FORGOTTEN HOME APOTHECARY II

Ancient Wisdom and Modern Applications for Healing

Stacy Lott

© 2024 Stacy Lott. All rights reserved.

Please note that unauthorized reproduction, storage, retrieval, transmission, or distribution of this publication is strictly prohibited without the publisher's prior written consent, as outlined in the 1976 US Copyright Act, Sections 107 and 108.

Limitation of Liability/Disclaimer of Warranty:

The publisher and the author provide no guarantees regarding the accuracy or completeness of the contents of this work. They specifically disclaim all warranties, including those related to fitness for a specific purpose. There are no warranties that can be created or extended through sales or promotional materials. Please note that the advice and strategies provided may not be suitable for all situations. This work is sold with the understanding that the publisher is not providing medical, legal, or other professional advice or services. If you need professional assistance, it is advisable to seek the services of a competent professional person. The publisher and author are not responsible for any damages that may occur. Please note that the inclusion of an individual, organization, or website as a citation or potential source of further information in this work does not imply endorsement by the author or publisher. The information or recommendations provided by these sources are not necessarily endorsed. Additionally, it is important for readers to note that any websites mentioned in this work may have undergone changes or become unavailable since the time of writing.

ISBN: 978-1-300-78318-3

Author: Stacy Lott

Book Title: Forgotten Home Apothecary II: Ancient Wisdom and Modern Applications for Healing

TABLE OF CONTENTS

INTRODUCTION	1
CHAPTER 1	4
HERBAL MEDICINE IN HISTORY	4
CHAPTER 2	10
THE SCIENCE BEHIND THE REMEDIES	10
CHAPTER 3	12
REMEDIES AND RECIPES	12
ABSCESS	13
FRESH YARROW POULTICE	13
ECHINACEA AND GOLDENSEAL TINCTURE	14
ACNE	16
CALENDULA TONER	16
AGRIMONY-CHAMOMILE GEL	17
ALLERGIES	19
FEVERFEW-PEPPERMINT TINCTURE	19
GARLIC-GINKGO SYRUP	20
ASTHMA	22
GINKGO-THYME TEA	22
PEPPERMINT-ROSEMARY VAPOR TREATMENT	23
ATHLETE'S FOOT	24
FRESH GARLIC POULTICE	24
GOLDENSEAL OINTMENT	25
BACKACHE	27
PASSIONFLOWER–BLUE VERVAIN TEA	27
GINGER-PEPPERMINT SALVE	28
BEE STING	30
FRESH PLANTAIN POULTICE	30

Comfrey-Aloe Gel	31
Bloating	**33**
Peppermint-Fennel Tea	33
Dandelion Root Tincture	34
Bronchitis	**35**
Rosemary–Licorice Root Vapor Treatment	35
Goldenseal-Hyssop Syrup	36
Bruise	**38**
Fresh Hyssop Poultice	38
Arnica Salve	39
Burn	**41**
Chickweed-Mullein Compress	41
Fresh Aloe Vera Gel	41
Canker Sore	**43**
Calendula-Comfrey Poultice	43
Goldenseal Tincture	44
Chapped Lips	**46**
Aloe-Calendula Balm	46
Comfrey-Hyssop Lip Balm	47
Chest Congestion	**49**
Hyssop-Sage Infusion	49
Angelica-Goldenseal Syrup	50
Chicken Pox	**52**
Comfrey-Licorice Bath	52
Calendula-Goldenseal Gel	53
Cold	**55**
Thyme Tea	55
Herbal Cold Syrup with Comfrey, Mullein, and Raspberry Leaf	56
Cold Sore	**58**
Garlic Poultice	58
Echinacea-Sage Toner	59
Conjunctivitis	**61**
Quick Chamomile Poultice	61
Goldenseal Poultice	62
Constipation	**63**
Aloe Vera Juice	63

Dandelion-Chickweed Syrup	64
Cough	**66**
Fennel-Hyssop Tea	66
Licorice-Thyme Cough Syrup	67
Dandruff	**69**
Echinacea Spray	69
Rosemary Conditioner	70
Diaper Rash	**71**
Chamomile-Echinacea Gel	71
Comfrey-Thyme Salve	72
Dry Skin	**74**
Chickweed-Aloe Gel	74
Calendula-Comfrey Body Butter	75
Earache	**77**
Blue Vervain Infusion and Poultice	77
Garlic-Mullein Infused Oil	78
Eczema	**80**
Calendula-Goldenseal Spray	80
Comfrey Salve	81
Fever	**83**
Feverfew Syrup	83
Blue Vervain–Raspberry Leaf Tincture	84
Flu	**86**
Catnip-Hyssop Tea	86
Garlic, Echinacea, and Goldenseal Syrup	87
Gingivitis	**89**
Calendula-Chamomile Mouth Rinse	89
Goldenseal-Sage Oil Pull	90
Hair Loss	**92**
Ginger Scalp Treatment	92
Ginkgo-Rosemary Tonic	93
Halitosis	**95**
Peppermint-Sage Mouthwash	95
Ginger-Mint Gunpowder Green Tea	96
Hangover	**98**
Feverfew-Hops Tea	98
Milk Thistle Tincture	99

HEADACHE	**101**
BLUE VERVAIN–CATNIP TEA	101
SKULLCAP TINCTURE	102
HEARTBURN	**104**
FRESH GINGER TEA	104
FENNEL-ANGELICA SYRUP	105
HIGH BLOOD PRESSURE	**106**
ANGELICA INFUSION	106
DANDELION-LAVENDER TINCTURE	107
INDIGESTION	**109**
CHAMOMILE-ANGELICA TEA	109
GINGER SYRUP	110
INSECT BITES	**111**
FRESH BASIL-MULLEIN SALVE	111
PEPPERMINT-PLANTAIN BALM	112
LARYNGITIS	**114**
MULLEIN-SAGE TEA	114
GINGER GARGLE	115
MENOPAUSE	**116**
FENNEL-SAGE DECOCTION	116
BLACK COHOSH TINCTURE	117
MENTAL WELLNESS	**118**
ST. JOHN'S WORT TEA	118
CHAMOMILE-PASSIONFLOWER DECOCTION	118
MUSCLE CRAMPS	**120**
ROSEMARY LINIMENT	120
GINGER SALVE	121
OILY SKIN	**123**
ROSEMARY TONER	123
PEPPERMINT SCRUB	124
PREMENSTRUAL SYNDROME (PMS)	**125**
DANDELION-GINGER TEA	125
BLACK COHOSH SYRUP	126
RINGWORM	**127**
FRESH GARLIC COMPRESS	127
GOLDENSEAL BALM	128
SORE MUSCLES	**130**

Ginger-Fennel Massage Oil	130
Peppermint–St. John's Wort Salve	131
Sore Throat	**133**
Peppermint Tea with Comfrey and Sage	133
Agrimony-Licorice Gargle	134
Sunburn	**135**
Comfrey Spray	135
Hyssop-Infused Aloe Vera Gel	136
Weight Loss	**137**
Dieter's Tea Blend with Chickweed, Dandelion, and Fennel	137
Ginseng Tincture	138

SECTION TWO 140

Key Herbs to Discover	140
Agrimony	141
Aloe	142
Angelica	143
Arnica	145
Basil	146
Black cohosh	147
Blue vervain	148
Catnip	150
Chamomile	151
Chickweed	152
Comfrey	153
Dandelion	155
Echinacea	156
Fennel	157
Feverfew	159
Garlic	160
Ginger	161
Ginkgo biloba	162
Goldenseal	163
Hops	164

MILK THISTLE	165
MULLEIN	166
PASSIONFLOWER	167
PEPPERMINT	168
RASPBERRY	169
ROSEMARY	170
SAGE	171
SAW PALMETTO	173
SKULLCAP	174
ST. JOHN'S WORT	175
THYME	176
TURMERIC	177
VALERIAN	178
WITCH HAZEL	179
YARROW	180
CONCLUSION	181

Introduction

Herbal medicine boasts a long and storied history, predating modern pharmaceuticals by thousands of years. Alternative medicine plays an important role and offers benefits in preventing and treating a range of common ailments.

Diverse herbs in the natural world possess incredible healing properties. With the right guidance and knowledge, anyone can harness the potential of herbs to relieve discomfort and promote healing.

Growing up in the mountains of Montana, I found fascination in the stories of Native Americans and their deep understanding of healing. They used the abundant wild plants near our home to craft remedies for different ailments. I became an adult and ventured into the world of teas beyond the usual peppermint and chamomile options. Today, I experience immense joy as I grow a diverse range of fragrant herbs in my garden and enjoy the beautiful hardwood forest that surrounds my home. I love exploring the great outdoors and taking leisurely walks through nature's wonders. Observing the diverse array of plants and their incredible healing properties captivates the mind. The soothing scents that fill the air enhance the experience. Whenever I don't feel my best, I rely on the plants I've harvested and prepared to boost my well-being.

Herbal remedies utilize plant parts in their fresh, natural form. Some people enjoy buying extracts from stores, while others take pleasure in making their own compounds at home. I have conducted thorough research and made thoughtful considerations to take charge of my well-being, successfully managing minor health issues before they escalate into serious conditions that require medical intervention. You can now try it out.

Buying medicinal herbs has become very easy, with pharmacies and large retail stores offering a wide range of options. Health food stores provide a diverse selection of whole herbs, tinctures, teas, ointments, and other products that serve as alternatives to pharmaceuticals.

Many conventional medications surprise people by tracing their roots back to herbal medicine.

Willow bark provides aspirin, and opium poppies yield morphine through careful extraction. Doctors obtain quinine, a crucial medication for treating malaria, from the bark of the cinchona tree. Doctors use digoxin, a potent medication, in cardiac cases. It comes from the beautiful yet poisonous foxglove plant. Researchers derive many pharmaceuticals from plants or synthesize them using compounds that closely resemble natural substances.

Conventional medicine often favors synthetic drugs due to their consistent formulations, purity, and convenience. Prescription pharmaceuticals have gained immense popularity. This book emphasizes their importance. It's important to remember that in the United States, regulators consider herbs as dietary supplements when sold commercially. When you choose a more holistic approach to healing, you don't need to obtain a prescription, unlike with synthetic medications. You can choose to use a herbal poultice, apply a basic cream or oil, or consume a tincture or tea.

Herbs pack a powerful punch, often lacking the long-term side effects that pharmaceuticals carry. Boosting the body's innate healing abilities, especially when paired with adequate rest, enhances our recovery potential. Various herbs boost the immune system, helping the body effectively utilize its natural defenses against viruses and infections.

Creating a complete list of medicinal plants presents an enormous task, and capturing the full range of properties displayed by each plant proves incredibly difficult. Choosing which herbs to use can be challenging with so many options available, despite the abundance of detailed guides out there.

This book stands out as exceptional. Discover a complete guide to harnessing the power of well-known and powerful medicinal herbs. Find all of them easily online or at a nearby health food store. You can likely find some of them thriving just a short distance from your home. A few might be lurking in your spice cabinet! This book serves as a valuable resource for those who are starting to explore herbal medicine or have already begun to appreciate the healing properties of plants.

Chapter I

Herbal Medicine in History

In the past, individuals sought natural remedies to address their health concerns, long before pharmaceutical companies emerged. Herbal medicine has evolved over time, whether through natural progression or trial and error, and it is not a recent development. Its resurgence stands out, particularly in light of the well-documented issues with conventional medications. Let's begin at the very start. Throughout history, various societies have harnessed the potential of their indigenous plants to create natural remedies. Diverse ecosystems on every continent provide a wide range of remedies tailored to the needs of various countries. Even in today's modern world, many individuals in different regions still face limited access to advanced medical treatments and medications. Herbal healers play a crucial role in public health.

Africa

Medicine has a rich history that spans thousands of years. Renowned scholars discovered the Edwin Smith Papyrus and Papyrus Ebers, which offer fascinating insights into ancient Egyptian medicine. Ancient works offer intricate descriptions of anatomy, meticulous records of injuries, and a wealth of knowledge on herbal pharmacology. They also create designs for medical and surgical instruments.

African traditional medicine values herbal remedies, utilizing around 4,000 indigenous plants from nature's pharmacy. African herbal medicines are gaining recognition from pharmaceutical companies. Local practitioners are currently collaborating and researching traditional remedies to identify bioactive agents for the creation of modern synthetic medicines.

Asia

Researchers discovered early literature on the use of Chinese herbs in Changsha, China, within the Mawangdui Han tombs sealed in 168 BCE. This comprehensive list of prescriptions, called Wushi'er Bingfang or Recipes for 52 Ailments, offers over 250 remedies for various health issues, including hemorrhoids and warts.

Traditional Asian medicine includes various practices such as massage, exercise, acupuncture, herbal treatments, and dietary therapy. China standardized these practices during the 1950s, but they have a rich history that dates back to about 1100 BCE, when numerous herbal remedies emerged.

By the end of the sixteenth century, traditional Asian physicians utilized a wide range of remedies. By the end of the twentieth century, the Chinese materia medica expanded significantly, including an impressive 12,800 different drugs.

The Atharva Veda in India served as a significant sourcebook, laying the foundation for Ayurveda, a healing practice dating back to around 1200 BCE. This system continues to be in use today.

Ancient Middle Eastern physicians shared their extensive knowledge of herbal medicine with scholars from Greece and Persia. Over time, Arabs shared their knowledge with European crusaders, who brought this invaluable information back to their countries.

Australia

In the 1600s, European ships first reached the shores of Australia. The true clash between indigenous and imperialist cultures occurred in 1788 when Britain's First Fleet arrived in Sydney, bringing around 1,500 individuals. Traditional communities in the past valued the use of herbal medicine highly.

However, their strong cultural tradition of oral history, which includes storytelling, singing, and dancing rituals, results in a lack of written records regarding Australia's earliest herbal medicines. The last practicing elders are passing away, decreasing the number of rituals and risking the loss of valuable knowledge about the continent's medicinal flora.

Today, people widely recognize traditional indigenous medicine as bush medicine. The practice focuses on traditional treatments that harness the healing properties of Australian leaves and seeds. People highly esteem indigenous remedies like native grapes and banksia flowers, while eucalyptus and turmeric have gained worldwide recognition for their exceptional qualities.

Europe

Early Greek and Roman physicians earned high regard for their vast understanding of herbs. Ancient Egyptian doctors passed down a considerable amount of their knowledge. Hippocrates, a trailblazer in medicine, learned from esteemed Egyptian priest-doctors.

After the fall of the Roman Empire, scientific progress stagnated, resulting in a notable decline in knowledge about herbal medicine. Increased trade with other civilizations sparked a resurgence in the exploration of medicinal herbs. During the Renaissance, European nobles dedicated themselves to gathering and systematizing a vast amount of knowledge in their libraries. They committed themselves to collecting the most valuable botanical specimens in their gardens. In the sixteenth and seventeenth centuries, universities offered courses on herbalism and botany, and they established "physic" gardens to cultivate medicinal plants.

Nicholas Culpeper published The English Physician in 1652, presenting a detailed compilation of herbal remedies found in England.

The author created the book for a broad audience, emphasizing the use of herbs for common ailments instead of expensive medical treatments.

In the modern era of science and technology, people have largely abandoned herbal remedies. Herbal remedies have regained popularity in Europe, overcoming the overshadowing of modern drugs.

North America

Throughout history, Native American and First Nations communities have recognized the value of natural remedies. They place great importance on holistic well-being to nurture the body, rejuvenate the spirit, and achieve mental harmony. Ancient oral traditions reveal that the earliest healers observed sick animals to understand medicinal herbs. Determining the historical usage of herbs by native North Americans before their contact with Europeans proves challenging due to the lack of written records. People primarily passed down the information through spoken stories. The situation shifted when indigenous people shared their natural remedies with the new settlers, who had knowledge of European herbal medicine. Many settlers brought their beloved medicinal plants with them as they traveled to the New World. These plants have spread across North America and grow alongside the continent's native flora.

Over time, European-style drugs gradually replaced traditional herbal remedies. In specific areas like Appalachia, Alaska, Hawaii, and remote tribal lands in the western United States and Canada, people actively use and trust herbal medicine as a common form of treatment.

South America

Indigenous populations of Central and South America extensively utilized medicinal plants. Modern practitioners actively engage in shamanic traditions, utilizing plant medicines that have held their esteemed reputation for centuries. This continent boasts a wealth of plants that offer a variety of medicinal properties. Local healers with a deep understanding of natural remedies often sell their products at market stalls. Forest workers often spend long periods in the jungle, using plants for sustenance, healing remedies, and materials to build shelters.

Isolated jungle areas hold truly astounding herbal knowledge. Ancient Mayan and Aztec healers possessed extensive knowledge of the healing properties of plants and actively utilized a wide range of treatments derived from them. They operated hospitals that provided specialized care and ensured patients remained separate from the rest of the population.

Today, cities, plantations, and ranches dominate the land in South America, leading to the loss of the once thriving native flora. The dense jungles of South America host a wide variety of medicinal plants. Researchers constantly discover exciting new species, highlighting the significance of conservation efforts and offering optimism for advancements in fields like malaria and cancer treatments.

Note

This book empowers individuals to take charge of their well-being and acknowledges the importance of modern medical treatment. Use caution and discretion when you utilize these treatments. Seek professional medical advice if you have a persistent medical condition.

Chapter 2

The Science Behind the Remedies

It has been found that a variety of herbs and botanicals form the basis for many commonly prescribed medications. As we explore the remedies, we'll delve deeper into this topic, but for now, let's provide a basic explanation of how herbal remedies work.

Optimal Digestive Health and Proper Liver Function

Natural remedies help treat common digestive issues like indigestion and nausea. A cup of peppermint or chamomile tea soothes and promotes relaxation.

Individuals who have experienced liver overload can find relief by incorporating specific herbs into their routine. These herbs protect and support the recovery process, helping to restore normal liver function after injury or illness.

Milk thistle supports liver health effectively.

Immune Function, Infection, and Inflammation

Various botanical medicines boost your immune system, support infection prevention, and reduce inflammation. Echinacea acts as a powerful herb that stimulates the immune system and helps prevent infections. Ginseng boosts the immune system and promotes overall well-being. People recognize St. John's wort, ginger, and ginkgo biloba for their strong anti-inflammatory properties.

Musculoskeletal Discomfort

Herbal medicines, both internal and external, can be highly effective in treating minor sprains, sore muscles, and painful joints. Plant-based ingredients with high antioxidant content can greatly benefit the maintenance of connective tissues. Herbs like calendula, witch hazel, and capsicum offer a soothing and comforting experience.

Psychological, Neurological, and Behavioral Health

When you see commercials for prescription drugs that claim to enhance mental well-being, it becomes clear that many of them come with cautionary notes about possible adverse reactions. Natural remedies like ginkgo biloba and valerian offer the potential to restore balance without any adverse effects.

Reproductive Health

Having knowledge about the right herbs can greatly assist in the management of premenstrual syndrome (PMS), menopause symptoms, and pregnancy side effects. Ginger has been found to be helpful in managing morning sickness, while black cohosh has been known to alleviate symptoms of both PMS and menopause. Certain herbs have been found to have potential benefits for supporting the male reproductive system. Examples include ginseng, ginkgo biloba, and saw palmetto.

Respiratory Health

Everyday health issues such as sore throats, coughs, and colds can be relieved with the assistance of easily accessible medications, although they may occasionally have undesirable side effects. However, these irritations can be successfully treated with herbal remedies, similar to how congested sinuses and mild respiratory infections are addressed. Echinacea is often utilized in remedies for cold and flu symptoms, while thyme and hyssop are recognized for their effectiveness in alleviating bronchial spasms and aiding in relaxation.

Chapter 3

Remedies and Recipes

Simple recipes, everyday kitchen tools, and a variety of herbal remedies effectively address common health issues. If you've experienced a bee sting while tending to your tomatoes or got hit by a flying baseball at your child's Little League game, you'll find a comprehensive list of helpful remedies here.

Abscess

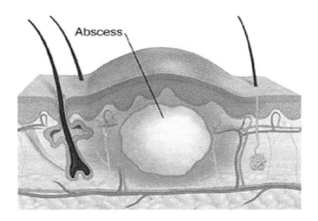

An abscess causes significant discomfort and feels warm to the touch. A region becomes inflamed or infected and fills with pus. An abscess grows larger, causing more severe discomfort. If natural remedies do not provide relief, consult a healthcare professional. An infection in a large abscess can spread to nearby tissue and even enter the bloodstream.

Fresh Yarrow Poultice

Makes 1 poultice

Yarrow has compounds that have anti-inflammatory and antibacterial properties. It has the ability to effectively eliminate bacteria, reduce inflammation, and speed up the healing process.

Ingredients

1 tablespoon of finely chopped fresh yarrow leaves.

Steps

Utilize the chopped leaves for the treatment of the abscess, ensuring that it is adequately covered with a gentle cloth. Leave the poultice in place for a duration of 10 to 15 minutes.

Keep up with this routine two or three times per day until the abscess is completely healed.

Precautions Do not use during pregnancy. Yarrow can cause skin reactions in people who are allergic to plants in the Asteraceae family.

Echinacea and Goldenseal Tincture

Makes about 2 cups

Echinacea and goldenseal have strong antibacterial properties and help boost the body's natural immune system. It's wise to prepare this tincture in advance for convenient access when necessary. When stored in optimal conditions, the quality of the product can be preserved for a duration of 7 years. Feel free to use it whenever you encounter an infection.

Ingredients

5 ounces dried echinacea root, finely chopped

3 ounces dried goldenseal root, finely chopped

2 cups unflavored 80-proof vodkatttt

Steps

Mix the echinacea and goldenseal in a clean pint jar. Make sure to add plenty of vodka, filling the jar to the brim and ensuring that the herbs are completely covered.

Ensure that the jar is tightly secured and vigorously shake it. Store it in a cool, dark cabinet and remember to give it a gentle shake every few days for 6 to 8 weeks. If any of the alcohol evaporates, be sure to add more vodka until the jar is filled to the brim again.

Place a moistened piece of cheesecloth over the opening of a funnel with caution. Pour the tincture into a fresh pint jar using the funnel. Squeeze the cheesecloth firmly to extract all the liquid from the roots. Get rid of the roots and transfer the finished tincture into dark glass bottles.

It is advised to take 10 drops orally two or three times a day for a duration of 7 to 10 days to treat an abscess..

Precautions Do not use during pregnancy. Use caution if you have diabetes, as goldenseal can sometimes lower blood sugar.

Acne

Red, inflamed, and infected sebaceous glands can cause painful pimples. This condition commonly affects teenagers, but adults can also experience it. Dealing with acne on your face or experiencing breakouts on your chest, back, or other parts of your body? Incorporate herbal remedies into your routine to enhance your appearance and promote a sense of well-being.

Calendula Toner

Makes about ½ cup

This gentle toner features calming calendula to help reduce inflammation and witch hazel to combat bacteria, leaving your skin feeling soft and refreshed. When stored in the ideal conditions, this toner will stay fresh for at least one year.

Ingredients

2 tablespoons calendula oil

⅓ cup witch hazel

Steps

Combine the ingredients in a glass bottle and give it a gentle shake.

Apply 5 or 6 drops to your clean face or any areas that need attention using a cotton cosmetic pad. Modify the quantity as needed.

Keep using twice daily until your acne clears up. If you're looking for a cool and refreshing experience, you might want to try storing the bottle in the refrigerator.

Agrimony-Chamomile Gel

Makes about ⅔ cup

When agrimony and chamomile are combined with aloe vera gel, they can effectively alleviate redness and inflammation. It is advised to keep the gel in the refrigerator. When properly stored in an airtight container, the product will maintain its freshness for a duration of two weeks.

Ingredients

2 teaspoons dried agrimony

2 teaspoons dried chamomile

½ cup water

¼ cup aloe vera gel

Steps

Mix the agrimony and chamomile together in a saucepan along with the water. Heat the mixture until it reaches a boiling point, then reduce the heat to a gentle simmer. Allow the mixture to simmer until it is reduced by half, then remove it from the heat and let it cool completely.

Wet a piece of cheesecloth and position it over the top of a funnel. Pour the mixture through the funnel into a glass bowl. Remove the liquid from the herbs by firmly squeezing the cheesecloth until all the liquid has been extracted.

Combine the aloe vera gel and liquid together using a whisk until thoroughly mixed. Place the completed gel into a fresh glass jar. Ensure that the jar is tightly sealed and stored in the refrigerator.

Apply a thin layer to the affected areas twice a day using a cotton cosmetic pad.

Precautions Omit the chamomile if you take prescription blood thinners or are allergic to plants in the ragweed family

Allergies

The immune system reacts unusually to common substances like cat dander, pollen, or dust, causing allergies. Avoiding allergens proves quite challenging since they appear in various sources like food, drinks, and the environment. Conventional treatments inhibit the immune response to allergens, while herbal remedies offer a milder alternative.

Feverfew-Peppermint Tincture

Makes about 2 cups

Using feverfew and peppermint can be beneficial in relieving symptoms during an allergy attack. If you'd rather steer clear of feverfew, you have the option of making a tincture using just peppermint. The tincture can be safely stored for up to 7 years in a cool, dark location.

Ingredients

2 ounces dried feverfew

6 ounces dried peppermint

2 cups unflavored 80-proof vodka

Steps

Mix the feverfew and peppermint in a clean pint jar. Please add the vodka, making sure that the jar is filled to its fullest.

Be sure to tightly seal the jar and give it a thorough shake. Store it in a cool, dark cabinet and remember to give it a gentle shake a few times each week for 6 to 8 weeks.

Wet a piece of cheesecloth and carefully position it over the top of a funnel. Pour the tincture into a fresh pint jar using the funnel.

Extract the liquid from the herbs. Properly discard the used herbs and transfer the finished tincture into glass bottles of a dark hue.

Take 5 drops orally as necessary when allergy symptoms occur. If the taste is too strong for your preference, you can choose to lessen it by blending it with a glass of water or juice before drinking.

Precautions Do not use feverfew if you are allergic to ragweed. Do not use feverfew during pregnancy.

Garlic-Ginkgo Syrup

Makes about 2 cups

Ginkgo biloba has natural antihistamine properties and offers various anti-inflammatory benefits, while garlic can help boost your immune system. If possible, choose honey that is sourced locally, as it may help boost your resistance to allergens in your area. This syrup will stay fresh for up to 6 months if kept in the refrigerator.

Ingredients

2 ounces fresh or freeze-dried garlic, chopped

2 ounces ginkgo biloba, crushed or chopped

2 cups water

1 cup local honey

Steps

Combine the garlic and ginkgo biloba with the water in a saucepan. Warm the liquid slowly until it begins to simmer, then partially cover with a lid and allow it to reduce by half.

Transfer the contents of the saucepan into a glass measuring cup. Next, carefully pour the mixture back into the saucepan using a piece of cheesecloth that has been slightly dampened. Continue squeezing the cheesecloth until all the liquid has been released.

Add the honey and heat the mixture on low, stirring constantly until it reaches a temperature of 105°F to 110°F.

Place the syrup into a sterilized container and store it in the refrigerator.

Consume 1 tablespoon orally three times a day until your allergy symptoms show signs of improvement.

Safety Measures Caution: Avoid use if you are currently taking a monoamine oxidase inhibitor (MAOI) for depression. It is important to consult with your doctor before using Ginkgo biloba, as it can potentially enhance the effects of blood thinners. For optimal results, it is recommended that children under the age of 12 take 1 teaspoon three times per day.

Asthma

Irritated airways throughout the lungs mark this condition, along with narrowed bronchial tubes. Difficulty breathing can frighten individuals and may trigger panic attacks.

Ginkgo-Thyme Tea

Makes 1 cup

If you're looking for natural ways to improve your breathing and promote relaxation in your chest muscles, you might want to try incorporating Ginkgo biloba and thyme into your routine. These herbs have been known to help open up airways and provide a sense of calm. If the taste of the tea isn't quite your cup of tea, you can always add a teaspoon of honey or dried peppermint to give it a more enjoyable flavor.

Ingredients

1 cup boiling water

1 teaspoon dried ginkgo biloba

1 teaspoon dried thyme

Steps

Fill a big mug with boiling water. Put in the dried herbs, cover the mug, and let the tea steep for 10 minutes. Take it easy and savor the tea while breathing in the steam. You can do this up to four times a day.

Peppermint-Rosemary Vapor Treatment

Makes 1 treatment

Peppermint helps open your airways and makes breathing easier, while rosemary leaves contain an oil that blocks histamine, offering benefits. If you don't have fresh herbs for this treatment, use 2 drops of peppermint essential oil and 4 drops of rosemary essential oil instead.

Ingredients

4 cups steaming-hot water (not boiling)

½ cup crushed fresh peppermint leaves

½ cup finely chopped fresh rosemary leaves

Steps

Mix together all the ingredients in a spacious, flat bowl. Place the bowl on a table and find a comfortable position in front of it.

Cover your head and the bowl with a large towel. Indulge in the captivating scent of the herbal vapors. Remember to take breaks when needed to get some fresh air. If you find the fumes overwhelming, just close your eyes for a moment. Continue the treatment until the water has cooled down.

Use as needed whenever asthma symptoms arise. You can use this treatment as often as you like, as it is gentle on your skin.

Athlete's Foot

A fungus thrives in damp, hot, and dim conditions, causing this unpleasant infection. Tackle the problem early to prevent it from spreading to your toenails. Untreated, it causes unattractive discoloration and disfigurement that proves difficult to eliminate.

Fresh Garlic Poultice

Makes 1 treatment

Garlic is a powerful antifungal agent that effectively treats athlete's foot. Utilizing raw honey can effectively combine the garlic with your feet, amplifying its antifungal properties. For optimal results, it is advised to prepare a new batch of this remedy for every treatment in order to enhance the healing process. Although it is possible to make a larger quantity and use it over a few days, using a fresh batch each time may lead to quicker results.

Ingredients

1 garlic clove, pressed

1 teaspoon raw honey

Steps

Mix the garlic and honey in a small bowl. Apply the blend to the affected area using a cotton cosmetic pad.

Put on a new pair of socks and relax for 15 minutes to an hour, letting the poultice do its thing. Be sure to thoroughly wash and dry your feet afterwards. Keep up with the treatment once or twice daily, and follow the instructions for applying Goldenseal Ointment. Continue for three days after symptoms have subsided.

Precautions Garlic may cause a skin rash in sensitive individuals.

Goldenseal Ointment

Makes about 1 cup

Goldenseal acts as a powerful antimicrobial agent that effectively combats athlete's foot. Choose to use this ointment on its own or boost its healing properties by combining it with a Fresh Garlic Poultice. The product stays fresh for up to a year when you store it properly.

Ingredients

1 cup light olive oil

2 ounces dried goldenseal root, chopped

1 ounce beeswax

Steps

Mix the olive oil and goldenseal in a slow cooker. Select the lowest heat setting, cover the slow cooker, and allow the roots to steep in the oil for 3 to 5 hours. Turn off the heat and allow the infused oil to cool down.

Heat a small amount of water until it reaches a gentle simmer in the base of a double boiler.

Reduce the heat to a lower setting.

Cover the upper portion of the double boiler with a piece of cheesecloth. Add the infused oil and firmly squeeze the cheesecloth to extract every last drop of oil. Get rid of the cheesecloth and herbs once you're done with them.

Mix the beeswax with the infused oil and place the double boiler on the base with caution.

Heat the mixture slowly over low heat. After the beeswax has fully melted, gently remove the pan from the heat source. Make sure to transfer the mixture into clean, dry jars or tins and allow it to cool completely before sealing.

Apply a small amount to the areas that require attention using a cotton cosmetic pad. Modify the quantity as needed and use up to three times a day, with the final application before going to sleep. It is advised to put on a fresh pair of socks over the ointment to avoid any possible slipping.

Precautions Do not use if you are pregnant or breastfeeding. Do not use if you have high blood pressure.

Backache

Back pain often arises from factors like overwork or injury, but it can also stem from inactivity, muscle spasms, or inflammation. Prioritize rest and relaxation to support your healing process. Encounter severe discomfort or notice any signs such as loss of sensation, tingling, or loss of bladder control? Seek advice from a medical professional immediately.

Passionflower–Blue Vervain Tea

Makes 1 cup

Passionflower and blue vervain have calming effects on the nervous system and can provide relief for tense muscles. This blend is incredibly soothing, so make sure to enjoy it when you have a moment to unwind.

Ingredients

1 cup boiling water

1 teaspoon dried passionflower

1 teaspoon dried blue vervain

Steps

Transfer the hot water into a spacious mug. Include the dried herbs, place a lid on the mug, and let the tea steep for 10 minutes. Take your time and savor the tea. Can be repeated up to two times daily

Precautions Do not use passionflower or blue vervain during pregnancy. Avoid passionflower if you have prostate problems or baldness.

Ginger-Peppermint Salve

Makes about 1 cup

Ginger and peppermint possess potent properties that can deeply penetrate the skin, inducing a soothing and comforting sensation that aids in muscle relaxation. This salve can maintain its freshness for up to a year when stored in a cool, dark place.

Ingredients

1 cup light olive oil

1 ounce dried gingerroot, chopped

1 ounce dried peppermint, crushed

1 ounce beeswax

Steps

Mix the olive oil, ginger, and peppermint in a slow cooker. Select the lowest heat setting, cover the slow cooker, and allow the herbs to steep in the oil for 3 to 5 hours. Turn off the heat and allow the infused oil to cool.

Heat a small amount of water until it reaches a gentle simmer in the base of a double boiler.

Reduce the heat to a gentle simmer.

Cover the upper part of the double boiler with a piece of cheesecloth. Once the infused oil is added, make sure to firmly squeeze the cheesecloth to ensure that every last drop of oil is extracted. Get rid of the cheesecloth and herbs once you're done with them.

Mix the beeswax with the infused oil and place the double boiler on the base with caution.

Gently heat over a low flame. After the beeswax has completely melted, gently remove the pan from the heat source. Make sure to transfer the mixture into clean, dry jars or tins and allow it to cool completely before sealing.

Use 1 teaspoon of the product and gently massage it into the affected area using your fingers or a cotton cosmetic pad. Modify the quantity as needed. Keep up with the treatment up to four times per day.

Bee Sting

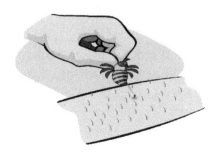

People often experience discomfort, inflammation, and swelling after a bee sting, and these symptoms can persist for a while. Herbs provide relief from discomfort. Herbal treatments offer benefits, but they cannot replace emergency EpiPens, particularly for those with a bee venom allergy.

Fresh Plantain Poultice

Makes 1 treatment

The plantain plant, distinct from the banana, is a green weed that contains aucubin, a powerful antitoxin.

Other components provide antiseptic and anti-inflammatory advantages, enhancing the effectiveness of this straightforward treatment. If fresh plantain leaves are not available, you can rehydrate a teaspoon of dried, crushed plantain in a tablespoon of water to use as a poultice.

Ingredients

1 tablespoon finely chopped fresh plantain leaves

Steps

Place the chopped leaves on the affected area and gently cover it with a soft cloth. Keep the poultice on for 10 to 15 minutes. Repeat as often as necessary until the pain subsides permanently.

Comfrey-Aloe Gel

Makes about ¼ cup

Comfrey possesses impressive anti-inflammatory and analgesic properties, offering soothing relief from the discomfort and inflammation resulting from bee stings. Aloe provides a calming effect and speeds up the recovery process. If you find this balm to your liking, you'll soon realize its versatility in treating various minor cuts and scrapes. When kept in the refrigerator, it stays fresh for about two weeks.

Ingredients

2 teaspoons dried comfrey

¼ cup water

2 tablespoons aloe vera gel

Steps

Combine the comfrey and water in a saucepan. Bring the mixture to a boil over high heat, then lower the heat to a gentle simmer. Cook the mixture until it reduces by half, then take it off the heat and let it cool completely.

Moisten a piece of cheesecloth and carefully place it over the opening of a funnel. Transfer the mixture through the funnel into a glass bowl. Extract the liquid from the comfrey by firmly squeezing the cheesecloth until all the liquid has been released.

Combine the aloe vera gel with the liquid and mix thoroughly using a whisk. Place the completed gel into a sterilized glass jar. Make sure to seal the jar securely and place it in the refrigerator.

Using a cotton cosmetic pad, gently apply a thin layer to the affected area whenever necessary until the pain and swelling decrease.

Bloating

Overeating, abdominal gas, and the onset of premenstrual cycles contribute to uncomfortable episodes of bloating. Herbs restore your body's balance by supporting the elimination of toxins, excess gas, and fluid buildup.

Peppermint-Fennel Tea

Makes 1 cup

If you think that your bloating may be due to buildup in your digestive tract, peppermint and fennel can offer you comfort and fast relief. These plants have a delightful taste and contain powerful antispasmodic agents that help to relax the smooth muscle tissue in the digestive tract. If the flavor of this tea is too strong for you, consider adding a teaspoon of honey.

Ingredients

1 cup boiling water

1 teaspoon dried peppermint

¼ teaspoon fennel seeds, crushed

Steps

Transfer the hot water into a spacious mug. Include the peppermint and fennel, place a lid on the mug, and let the tea steep for 10 minutes.

Take a moment to unwind and savor your cup of tea. This remedy is gentle and can be used as frequently as necessary.

Dandelion Root Tincture

Makes about 2 cups

Dandelion root has a bitter taste, but it provides potent diuretic benefits that can aid in the elimination of toxins and promote a greater sense of comfort. This tincture can maintain its freshness for a remarkable 7 years when stored in a cool, dark place.

Ingredients

8 ounces dandelion root, finely chopped

2 cups unflavored 80-proof vodka

Steps

Put the dandelion root in a clean pint jar. Make sure to add a generous amount of vodka, filling the jar to its maximum capacity and ensuring that the roots are completely submerged.

Ensure that the jar is tightly sealed and give it a thorough shake. Store it in a cool, dark cabinet and remember to give it a gentle shake a few times each week for 6 to 8 weeks. If any of the alcohol evaporates, just add more vodka to fill the jar to the brim once again.

Take a piece of cheesecloth and gently position it over the opening of a funnel, making sure it is damp. Pour the tincture into a fresh pint jar using the funnel. Squeeze the cheesecloth firmly to extract all the liquid from the roots. Make sure to properly discard the roots and carefully transfer the finished tincture into dark glass bottles.

Consume 1 teaspoon orally once or twice per day when experiencing bloating. If the taste is too strong for your preference, you can choose to lessen it by diluting it with a glass of water or juice before drinking.

Bronchitis

Irritation, infection, or allergies often lead to bronchitis, causing inflammation of the bronchial linings. A deep, rasping cough often characterizes the condition. Natural remedies, along with a commitment to staying hydrated and getting enough rest, effectively relieve and eliminate the symptoms of bronchitis.

Rosemary–Licorice Root Vapor Treatment

Makes 1 treatment

Rosemary and licorice root can assist in opening the airways, promoting circulation, and providing relief from the discomfort and inflammation commonly associated with bronchitis.

Ingredients

5 cups water

¼ cup chopped dried licorice root

½ cup finely chopped fresh rosemary leaves

Steps

Mix the water and dried licorice root in a saucepan. Bring the mixture to a boil, then reduce the heat. Simmer the mixture for 10 minutes.

Mix the water and licorice root in a shallow bowl, then add the rosemary leaves.

Cover your head and the bowl with a generously-sized towel. Breathe in the delightful aromas that softly drift from the herbs. Remember to take breaks when needed to get some fresh air. If the environment becomes overwhelming, just close your eyes for a moment. Continue the treatment until the water has cooled down.

Continue as needed. This treatment can be used as often as you like without any negative effects.

Precautions Do not use this treatment if you have epilepsy, high blood pressure, diabetes, kidney problems, or heart disease.

Goldenseal-Hyssop Syrup

Makes about 2 cups

Goldenseal is known for its powerful antiviral and antibacterial properties, thanks to the presence of hydrastine and berberine. Hyssop is known for its ability to alleviate bronchial spasms and promote the clearance of lung congestion. Additionally, it has a soothing and calming effect that can assist in relaxation. This syrup is also effective in treating the common cold. It can be stored in the refrigerator for up to 6 months.

Ingredients

½ ounce dried goldenseal root, chopped

1 ounce dried hyssop

2 cups water

1 cup honey

Steps

Mix the goldenseal and hyssop together with the water in a saucepan. Warm the liquid slowly until it begins to simmer, then partially cover with a lid and allow it to reduce by half.

Transfer the contents of the saucepan into a glass measuring cup, and strain the mixture through a dampened piece of cheesecloth back into the saucepan. Press the cheesecloth firmly to ensure all the liquid is fully extracted.

Combine the honey and heat the mixture over low heat, stirring constantly until it reaches a temperature of 105°F to 110°F.

Place the syrup into a sterilized jar or bottle and store it in the refrigerator.

Administer 1 tablespoon orally three to five times per day until your symptoms improve.

Precautions: It is not recommended to use this product during pregnancy or while breastfeeding. Warning: Individuals with epilepsy or high blood pressure should exercise caution. Goldenseal can potentially exacerbate symptoms of diarrhea and heartburn. For children under age 12, it is advised to take 1 teaspoon two to three times per day.

Bruise

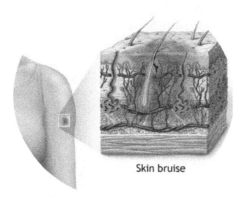
Skin bruise

Deep, painful bruises can indicate the existence of additional injuries or health complications. Accidental contact with objects can sometimes lead to minor bruises. If you happen to observe a rise in the frequency of bruising, it would be wise to seek advice from a medical professional, as this may be a sign of an underlying health issue.

Fresh Hyssop Poultice

Makes 1 treatment

Hyssop provides pain relief and promotes circulation, which can accelerate the healing process of your bruise. If you haven't already incorporated hyssop into your garden, you can utilize a small amount of hyssop essential oil to address a bruise. Another option is to rehydrate a teaspoon of dried hyssop with a tablespoon of warm water and use it to make a poultice.

Ingredients

1 tablespoon finely chopped fresh hyssop leaves

Steps

Place the chopped leaves on the affected area and gently cover it with a soft cloth. Keep the poultice in place for 10 to 15 minutes.

Continue this routine two or three times daily until the bruise gradually disappears.

Precautions Hyssop can produce sudden and involuntary muscle contractions, so it should not be used if you have epilepsy or are pregnant.

Arnica Salve

Makes about 1 cup

Arnica is a powerful anti-inflammatory agent, and its pain-relieving properties make this simple salve a great option for bumps and bruises.

Ingredients

1 cup light olive oil

2 ounces dried arnica flowers

1 ounce beeswax

Steps

Mix the olive oil and arnica in a slow cooker. Opt for the lowest heat setting, ensure the slow cooker is covered, and allow the herbs to steep in the oil for a duration of 3 to 5 hours. Turn off the heat and allow the infused oil to cool down.

Warm a small amount of water in the base of a double boiler until it begins to simmer.

Reduce the heat to a lower setting.

Position a layer of cheesecloth delicately on top of the upper portion of the double boiler. After adding the infused oil, make sure to squeeze the cheesecloth tightly to extract every last drop of oil. Get rid of the cheesecloth and herbs once you're done with them.

Mix the beeswax with the infused oil and place the double boiler on the base with caution.

Gently heat over a low flame. After the beeswax has fully melted, cautiously remove the pan from the heat source. Transfer the mixture into clean, dry jars or tins and allow it to cool completely before sealing.

Apply a small amount to the affected area using your fingers or a cotton cosmetic pad. Modify the quantity as needed and use it two times a day until the bruise fades away.

Precautions: Do not use on broken skin. Irritation can occur with long-term use; discontinue if signs of skin irritation appear.

Burn

Natural remedies effectively treat minor burns, like those that occur during cooking. Immediately seek medical attention for burns that appear severe, with charred skin or extensive coverage on the body.

Chickweed-Mullein Compress

Makes 1 treatment

Mullein has properties that can help prevent burns from getting infected and provide relief from pain.

Chickweed offers an extra level of cooling and aids in expediting the healing process.

Ingredients

2 teaspoons finely chopped chickweed

1 teaspoon finely chopped fresh mullein leaf

Steps

Apply the freshly cut plant material to the burn and the area around it, then cover it with a gentle cloth. Keep the poultice on for 10 to 15 minutes. Continue the repetition every 2 to 3 hours or more frequently, until the pain diminishes.

Fresh Aloe Vera Gel

Makes 1 treatment

Aloe vera gel has powerful antibacterial properties that effectively protect burns from infection. Additionally, it provides soothing anti-inflammatory benefits. Aloe has the ability to stimulate collagen synthesis, which can help accelerate the regeneration process of the skin following a minor burn. Although it is most effective when used immediately after being extracted from the plant, bottled aloe gel can be a suitable alternative.

Ingredients

Aloe vera plant

Steps

Take a 1-inch section from the tip of an aloe vera leaf. Keep the remaining leaf on the plant to support its ongoing growth.

Using a precise knife, carefully cut the leaf open. Apply the gel from the center of the leaf to the burn and the surrounding area using your fingers or a cotton cosmetic pad. Make sure to repeat this process once or twice a day while your burn is healing.

Canker Sore

A canker sore, a bothersome red blister that appears in the mouth, can be quite annoying, but it usually doesn't warrant concern. If canker sores occur frequently, seek guidance from a healthcare professional, as they could indicate an underlying metabolic disorder.

Calendula-Comfrey Poultice

Makes 1 treatment

Calendula is known for its soothing properties and ability to promote faster healing of minor wounds. It also has antifungal, anti-inflammatory, and antibacterial benefits. Comfrey is known for its healing properties and can provide some relief from the pain and itching associated with canker sores. If you enjoy this treatment, you can optimize your time by creating multiple dry poultices simultaneously.

Ingredients

⅛ teaspoon dried calendula

⅛ teaspoon dried comfrey

2 tablespoons hot water

Steps

Utilize a mortar and pestle or grinder to finely grind the herbs, then carefully transfer the resulting powder onto a small piece of muslin fabric.

Carefully fold the muslin into a compact packet, making sure to enclose the fragrant herbs. Immerse it in hot water for 2 minutes.

Insert the completed poultice into your mouth, ensuring that the fabric layer is thin and in contact with the canker sore. Keep it in place for 10 to 15 minutes. Repeat the process two or three times per day until the canker sore is gone.

Goldenseal Tincture

Makes about ⅔ cup

Goldenseal root contains high levels of berberine and hydrastine, providing it with a broad spectrum of antiviral and antibacterial properties, which makes it a valuable herb. This goldenseal tincture effectively treats canker sores and also works well for minor cuts, scrapes, and burns.

You can also take it internally if you feel the symptoms of a cold or the flu coming on.

Ingredients

4 ounces dried goldenseal root, finely chopped

1 cup unflavored 80-proof vodka

Steps

Place the goldenseal in a sanitized half-pint jar. Fill the jar to the brim with vodka, ensuring that the roots are completely covered.

Make sure to seal the jar securely and give it a good shake. Keep it in a cool, dark cabinet and give it a good shake a few times each week for 6 to 8 weeks. If any of the alcohol evaporates, make sure to replenish it with more vodka until the jar is filled to the brim once again.

Moisten a piece of cheesecloth and carefully place it over the opening of a funnel. Transfer the tincture through the funnel into a clean, sterilized half-pint jar. Extract the liquid from the roots by firmly squeezing the cheesecloth until all the liquid has been wrung out. Remove the roots and carefully transfer the completed tincture into glass bottles that are dark in color.

Apply 2 or 3 drops on the canker sore using a cotton swab. Inhale through your mouth to prevent excessive saliva while the tincture dries. Continue using this method two or three times per day until the canker sore goes away.

Precautions: Not recommended for use during pregnancy or while breastfeeding. Do not use if you have high blood pressure.

Chapped Lips

Lips sometimes crack, roughen, or peel, leading to discomfort that extends beyond a cosmetic issue. When the lips cannot naturally produce moisture, dryness often occurs.

Environmental factors like sun, wind, heating, and air-conditioning can worsen the situation. Licking your lips may seem like a way to moisturize them, but it can actually worsen the discomfort instead of providing relief.

Aloe-Calendula Balm

Makes 2 tablespoons

Aloe vera and calendula are beneficial for healing compromised skin, while aloe provides much-needed moisture to dry lips. This recipe utilizes a ready-made calendula oil, but feel free to substitute it with your own homemade infused calendula oil. When properly stored, this balm will remain fresh for up to a year.

Ingredients

1½ tablespoons aloe vera gel

1½ teaspoons calendula oil

Steps

Combine the aloe vera gel and calendula oil in a small bowl. Make sure to blend them thoroughly with a whisk.

Move the balm to a container that has a secure lid. If you want to ensure the freshness of your main supply, it's recommended to keep it refrigerated. However, you may also consider carrying a small squeeze bottle with a teaspoon of it to conveniently apply throughout the day.

Using either your fingertip or a cotton swab, gently apply a thin layer to your lips. Only a small amount is necessary, apply as necessary during the day and before going to sleep.

Comfrey-Hyssop Lip Balm

Makes about ⅔ cup (enough to fill 10 lip balm tubes)

Comfrey and hyssop possess properties that can effectively alleviate inflammation and pain, thereby accelerating the healing of damaged skin and providing relief from the discomfort of chapped lips. This recipe can be easily adapted to accommodate different serving sizes. The final product can maintain its freshness for about one year when stored in a cool, dark place.

Ingredients

2 tablespoons jojoba oil

1 tablespoon cocoa butter

1 tablespoon light olive oil

1 teaspoon dried comfrey

1 teaspoon dried hyssop

4 teaspoons grated beeswax or beeswax pastilles

3 drops vitamin E oil (optional)

Steps

Heat a small amount of water until it reaches a gentle simmer in the base of a double boiler.

Reduce the heat to a low setting.

Mix together the jojoba oil, cocoa butter, olive oil, and herbs in a glass measuring cup. Place the measuring cup in the upper part of the double boiler and allow it to heat gradually over low heat for a period of 2 to 3 hours. Make sure to keep an eye on the water level in the base of the double boiler to avoid any possible evaporation.

Set up a small bowl and use a piece of cheesecloth to cover it. Strain the infused oil into the bowl with care. Thoroughly squeeze and wring the cheesecloth to ensure complete extraction of the oil.

Get rid of the cheesecloth and herbs once you're done with them.

Put the infused oil back into the measuring cup and mix in the beeswax. Put the measuring cup back on the double boiler and gently heat it over low heat until the beeswax has melted, making sure not to use excessive heat.

Remove the measuring cup from the double boiler and add the vitamin E oil, if you prefer. Transfer the mixture into empty lip balm tubes or tins and allow it to cool completely before sealing.

For the best results, it's important to apply a thin layer of balm to your lips throughout the day and before going to bed.

Precautions: Omit the hyssop and double the comfrey if you are pregnant or have epilepsy.

Chest Congestion

If you're having trouble with your breathing, herbs can help alleviate lung discomfort and improve your overall comfort while you address the root cause of your congestion.

Hyssop-Sage Infusion

Makes 1 quart

Hyssop has powerful antiviral properties and is known for its effectiveness as an expectorant. Sage has beneficial antiseptic properties that can aid in faster healing. This blend offers a robust herbal flavor that appeals to certain individuals, while others may prefer to enhance its palatability by adding a touch of honey.

Ingredients

4 cups boiling water

4 teaspoons dried hyssop

4 teaspoons dried sage

Steps

Combine the boiling water and dried herbs in a teapot. Cover the pot and let the infusion steep for 10 minutes.

Take a moment to unwind and savor the soothing aroma as you leisurely sip on your infusion. You have the option to reheat or refrigerate the remaining portion and enjoy it throughout the day.

Angelica-Goldenseal Syrup

Makes about 2 cups

Angelica relieves congestion by gently stimulating and warming the lungs, providing relief from associated discomfort. Goldenseal possesses powerful antiseptic and antiviral properties that help speed up your recovery from illness. Honey soothes your throat and masks the strong flavors, especially if you feel irritation from coughing. Store this syrup in the refrigerator to keep it fresh for up to 6 months.

Ingredients

1 ounce angelica, finely chopped

1 ounce dried goldenseal root, finely chopped

2 cups water

1 cup honey

Steps

Combine the herbs and water in a saucepan. Simmer the liquid over low heat, partially covering it with a lid, until it is reduced by half.

Transfer the contents of the saucepan to a glass measuring cup, then pour the mixture through a dampened piece of cheesecloth back into the saucepan, squeezing the cheesecloth until no more liquid is extracted.

Include the honey and gently heat the mixture on a low flame, stirring continuously until the temperature reaches 105°F to 110°F.

Transfer the syrup to a sterilized jar or bottle and keep it in the refrigerator.

Take 1 tablespoon orally three or four times per day until your symptoms improve. For children under age 12, it is recommended to take 1 teaspoon two or three times per day.

Chicken Pox

Chicken pox causes a highly infectious rash that irritates and fills with fluid-filled blisters. While no known cure exists for chicken pox, you can incorporate herbal remedies into your routine to alleviate discomfort.

Comfrey-Licorice Bath

Makes 1 quart

Comfrey and licorice root provide relief for the itching caused by chicken pox and also have antiviral properties. The apple cider vinegar has a strong aroma, but it enhances the soothing effect. This simple recipe utilizes pre-made comfrey and licorice root tinctures, although you have the option to substitute them with your own homemade versions.

Ingredients

4 cups organic unfiltered apple cider vinegar

½ teaspoon comfrey tincture

½ teaspoon licorice root tincture

Steps

Combine the vinegar and tinctures in a clean, dry jar. Seal tightly and keep in a cool, dark place until you're ready to use it.

Prepare a warm bath and add 1 cup of the mixture to the water. Make sure to spend at least 20 minutes soaking. Make sure to repeat once or twice per day.

Precautions: Do not use licorice root if you have high blood pressure, diabetes, kidney problems, or heart disease.

Calendula-Goldenseal Gel

Makes about 2 cups

Aloe, calendula, and goldenseal work together to soothe itching and irritation from chicken pox blisters, actively supporting the healing process. This gel effectively addresses a wide range of skin conditions, including rashes, irritations, and minor cuts and scrapes. The refrigerator keeps the product fresh for up to 2 weeks.

Ingredients

1 ounce dried calendula

1 ounce dried goldenseal root, chopped

2 cups water

1½ cups aloe vera gel

Steps

Mix the calendula and goldenseal together with the water in a saucepan. Heat the mixture until it comes to a boil, then reduce the heat to a gentle simmer.

Continue cooking the mixture until only about ½ cup remains, then remove it from the stove and allow it to cool completely.

Dampen a piece of cheesecloth and gently position it over the top of a funnel. Pour the mixture into a glass bowl using the funnel. Squeeze the cheesecloth firmly to extract all the liquid from the herbs.

Mix the aloe vera gel with the liquid using a whisk. Put the finished gel in a glass jar that has been sterilized. Ensure that the jar is tightly sealed and stored in the refrigerator.

Apply a thin layer to the affected areas two or three times a day using a cotton cosmetic pad.

Cold

Coughing, sneezing, and a sore throat can really disrupt your day. Treat your cold as soon as symptoms appear to reduce its duration.

Thyme Tea

Makes 1 cup

Thyme has the ability to act as an antitussive, which means it can effectively suppress coughing and provide quick relief. It serves a dual purpose by helping to clear congestion from the lungs as an expectorant. Additionally, it provides relief for a sore throat and alleviates the body aches commonly experienced with a cold. If you prefer a sweeter flavor, you can add a teaspoon of honey to this tea.

Ingredients

1 cup boiling water

2 teaspoons dried thyme

Steps

Transfer the hot water into a spacious mug. Include the thyme, place a lid on the mug, and let the tea steep for 10 minutes.

Take your time and savor the tea as you enjoy the soothing aroma. Repeat up to six times per day.

Herbal Cold Syrup with Comfrey, Mullein, and Raspberry Leaf

Makes about 2 cups

Comfrey has potential benefits for coughs and sore throats, while mullein, thyme, and raspberry leaf possess properties that may assist with fever, body aches, and lung irritation. It's not a problem if you don't have all the herbs for this recipe. All of these have properties that can be helpful in relieving your cold symptoms. The syrup can stay fresh for up to 6 months if kept in the refrigerator.

Ingredients

½ ounce dried comfrey

½ ounce dried mullein

½ ounce dried raspberry leaf

½ ounce dried thyme

2 cups water

1 cup honey

Steps

Mix the herbs and water in a saucepan. Allow the liquid to gently simmer over low heat, partially covering it with a lid, until it is reduced by half.

Transfer the contents of the saucepan into a glass measuring cup. Next, carefully pour the mixture back into the saucepan using a piece of cheesecloth that has been slightly dampened. Press the cheesecloth firmly to ensure all the liquid is extracted.

Add the honey and warm the mixture on low heat, stirring constantly until it reaches a temperature of 105°F to 110°F.

Place the syrup in a sterilized jar or bottle and store it in the refrigerator to keep it chilled.

Administer 1 tablespoon orally, three or four times daily, until your symptoms show signs of improvement. For best results, it is suggested that children who are younger than 12 years old consume 1 teaspoon two or three times daily.

Precautions: Never use raspberry leaves that are not completely dried, as fresh ones can cause nausea

Cold Sore

The herpes simplex virus causes cold sores that commonly appear in the mouth and on the lips. Consider using herbal remedies at the first signs of tingling or itching, before blister clusters form.

An untreated cold sore can allow the virus to spread, and herbal remedies might not be strong enough to stop it. They provide soothing comfort.

Garlic Poultice

Makes 1 treatment

Despite its pungent odor, raw garlic is known for its potent antiviral properties that may help shorten the duration of a cold sore. If you don't want to go through the hassle of holding the garlic in place, you could try using a piece of first aid tape to secure it. This way, you can get multiple tasks done at once.

Ingredients

1 garlic clove, cut in half

Steps

Make sure to wash and dry the affected area thoroughly.

Place the cut side of the garlic on the cold sore and keep it there for 10 minutes. Continue this routine three or four times daily until the cold sore disappears.

Precautions: Garlic can cause a skin rash in sensitive individuals; discontinue treatment if this occurs.

Echinacea-Sage Toner

Makes about ½ cup

Echinacea and sage provide powerful antiviral and antibacterial properties, which can effectively prevent the sores from getting infected. The witch hazel and aloe are effective in providing relief from itching. This toner has a long shelf life of at least one year when stored in a refrigerator.

Ingredients

½ ounce dried echinacea root, chopped

½ ounce dried sage, crumbled

2 tablespoons jojoba or light olive oil

2 tablespoons aloe vera gel

¼ cup witch hazel

Steps

Combine the herbs and oil in a slow cooker. Choose the lowest heat setting, cover the slow cooker, and let the herbs steep in the oil for 3 to 5 hours.

Switch off the heat and let the infused oil cool down.

Place a piece of cheesecloth gently over a bowl. Strain the infused oil using the cheesecloth, making sure to squeeze out every last drop. Dispose of the cheesecloth and used herbs.

Place the infused oil into a glass bottle of a darker hue, and proceed to incorporate the aloe vera gel and witch hazel. Mix the ingredients by shaking gently.

Using a cotton swab, gently apply a small amount to the area that needs attention. Adjust the amount as necessary.

Continue using this method two or three times daily until the cold sore goes away. It is recommended to keep the bottle in the refrigerator.

Precautions: Omit the echinacea if you are allergic to ragweed or have an autoimmune disease.

Conjunctivitis

Redness, itching, crusting or discharge, and tearing of the eyes commonly signal conjunctivitis. Pinkeye, a common issue, causes dry eyes, swollen eyelids, and increased sensitivity to light.

Quick Chamomile Poultice

Makes 1 treatment

Chamomile is known for its soothing properties that can help alleviate the discomfort and irritation caused by conjunctivitis. It also has anti-inflammatory and antibacterial properties, making it a beneficial treatment option. Using plain chamomile tea bags, preferably organic, is a convenient and straightforward way to utilize this remedy when you're in a hurry.

Ingredients

¼ cup steaming-hot (not boiling) water

1 organic chamomile tea bag

Steps

Place the water in a small cup or bowl and immerse the tea bag in it. Let it sit for 2 minutes.

Take out the tea bag from the water and let it cool down until it reaches a temperature that is warm and pleasant to touch. Take a moment to close your eye and find a state of relaxation. Gently press the tea bag against your eye and let it sit for 10 to 20 minutes. Replace two or three times per day while recovering from conjunctivitis.

Goldenseal Poultice

Makes 1 treatment

Goldenseal is highly effective in treating conjunctivitis due to its soothing properties that help reduce irritation, fight inflammation, and combat infection. If you enjoy this method, you can streamline the process by preparing multiple poultices ahead of time and simply activating them with hot water when you're ready to apply them.

Ingredients

½ cup steaming-hot water (not boiling)

1 tablespoon chopped dried goldenseal root

Steps

Transfer the hot water into a small bowl. Place the chopped goldenseal root in a reusable linen bag and submerge the bag in the hot water. Let the poultice soak in the water for 5 to 10 minutes, or until the roots become soft.

Take a moment to close your eyes and find a state of relaxation. Gently apply the poultice to your eye and let it sit for 10 to 20 minutes. Make sure to repeat two or three times per day while recovering from conjunctivitis.

Constipation

People often experience abdominal discomfort and difficulties with bowel movements due to constipation. Herbs offer a gentle and effective way to find relief, eliminating the need for harsh chemical laxatives. Incorporate more fiber into your diet, stay properly hydrated, and engage in regular physical activity to boost your productivity.

Aloe Vera Juice

Makes about 3 cups

Aloe vera juice enhances digestion and effectively cleanses the digestive tract. This makes it ideal for addressing long-term constipation issues. It is recommended to consume freshly made aloe juice within 3 days.

Ingredients

1 fresh 3-to 4-inch aloe leaf from the inner portion of the plant

3 cups fresh juice, water, or coconut water

Steps

Flip the aloe leaf over the sink to let the resin drain away from the cut. Once the resin has stopped dripping, slice the leaf in half vertically and gently extract the gel from the interior. Transfer the gel to a blender and pour in the liquid. Blend thoroughly, refrigerate, and savor the refreshing result. Consume 1 cup daily and store any remaining mixture in a tightly sealed container in the refrigerator.

Dandelion-Chickweed Syrup

Makes about 2 cups

Both dandelion and chickweed are effective natural remedies for relieving constipation, offering a gentle alternative to harsh chemicals. You may be able to find both of these herbs in your own backyard. Just ensure that they haven't been contaminated with herbicide or chemical fertilizer. This syrup can stay fresh for up to 6 months if stored in the refrigerator.

Ingredients

1 ounce dandelion root, chopped

1 ounce fresh or dried chickweed

2 cups water

1 cup honey

Steps

Mix the dandelion root, chickweed, and water in a saucepan. Bring the liquid to a gentle simmer over low heat, partially covering it with a lid, and let the liquid reduce by half.

Transfer the contents of the saucepan into a glass measuring cup, and strain the mixture back into the saucepan using a dampened piece of cheesecloth. Press the cheesecloth firmly to ensure all the liquid is fully extracted.

Combine the honey and heat the mixture over a low flame, making sure to stir constantly until it reaches a temperature of 105°F to 110°F.

Place the syrup in a sterilized jar or bottle and store it in the refrigerator.

Take one tablespoon orally three or four times a day until your symptoms improve. For children under age 12, it is advised to take 1 teaspoon two or three times per day.

Cough

Coughing is a normal physiological reaction that aids in the expulsion of irritants and excess phlegm from the respiratory system. Beginning as a bothersome tickle in your throat, this can progress into a more severe and persistent cough that is dry and unproductive. Natural remedies can be beneficial in providing relief for irritated throat tissues while you focus on resolving the underlying issue.

Fennel-Hyssop Tea

Makes 1 cup

Fennel helps to loosen phlegm, which can make coughs more productive. If you're experiencing a dry, hacking cough and an irritated throat, you'll be pleased to know that this tea contains fennel and hyssop, which can provide fast relief from the discomfort.

Ingredients

1 cup boiling water

1 teaspoon fennel seeds

1 teaspoon dried hyssop

Steps

Transfer the hot water into a spacious mug. Add the herbs, cover the mug, and let the tea steep for 10 minutes.

Take your time and savor the tea as you enjoy the soothing steam. Can be repeated up to four times per day.

Licorice-Thyme Cough Syrup

Makes about 2 cups

Using licorice root can effectively reduce inflammation in the throat, providing fast relief for irritated tissue. Thyme, on the other hand, acts as an expectorant, helping to clear the lungs.

Thyme is also known for its antitussive properties, helping to soothe coughing spasms. This cough syrup has a shelf life of 6 months when stored in the refrigerator.

Ingredients

1 ounce licorice root, chopped

1 ounce thyme

2 cups water

1 cup honey

Steps

Mix the licorice root, thyme, and water in a saucepan. Warm the liquid slowly until it begins to simmer, then partially cover it with a lid and allow it to reduce by half.

Transfer the contents of the saucepan into a glass measuring cup. Next, carefully pour the mixture back into the saucepan by filtering it through a moistened cheesecloth, ensuring that all the liquid is extracted.

Combine the honey and heat the mixture over a low flame, making sure to stir constantly until it reaches a temperature of 105°F to 110°F.

Pour the syrup into a clean jar or bottle and store it in the fridge.

Take one tablespoon orally three or four times daily until your symptoms show improvement. To achieve the best possible outcomes, it is advised that children who are younger than 12 years old consume 1 teaspoon of the product two or three times daily.

Dandruff

Dandruff sometimes results from a fungal infection or scalp psoriasis, causing an itchy and flaky scalp. However, it often responds well to mild herbal remedies.

Echinacea Spray

Makes about 1 cup

Echinacea effectively combats candida, a common culprit in severe cases of dandruff, while witch hazel provides relief from the persistent itching. If your scalp is damaged from itching, the witch hazel will help it heal. This spray can remain fresh for up to a year when stored in the refrigerator.

Ingredients

1 cup witch hazel

2 tablespoons echinacea tincture

Steps

Mix the ingredients in a stylish glass bottle equipped with a spray top.

Shake gently to ensure thorough blending.

Apply 1 or 2 spritzes to each part of your scalp where you're experiencing dandruff.

Apply the spray with care, using your fingertips, and then brush or comb your hair. You can choose to style your hair as you usually do and leave the spray in all day if you prefer. Alternatively, you can opt to rinse it out with shampoo after 1 to 2 hours. For best results, use daily.

Important Safety Measures: It is important to exercise caution when considering the use of echinacea, especially if you have an autoimmune disorder or are allergic to ragweed.

Rosemary Conditioner

Makes 1 cup

This straightforward antifungal remedy combines a natural, unscented conditioner tailored to your specific hair type with rosemary essential oil, which is highly concentrated and delightfully fragrant. If you don't happen to have rosemary essential oil on hand, you can easily substitute it with tincture.

Ingredients

1 cup natural, unscented herbal conditioner like Stonybrook Botanicals

40 drops rosemary essential oil

Steps

Combine the conditioner and essential oil in a large bowl, ensuring they are thoroughly blended using a whisk or fork. Transfer it to a BPA-free plastic bottle with a squeeze top using a funnel.

After shampooing, apply a dollop of conditioner to your scalp, adjusting the amount as necessary to ensure full coverage. Wait for 2 to 5 minutes, then rinse the conditioner out with cool water. Style your hair as you normally would. For optimal results, use on a daily basis.

Diaper Rash

Diaper rash may occasionally occur, even with diligent diaper changes. It may result in discomfort, inflammation, and edema. Natural remedies are ideal for your baby's sensitive skin, as they do not contain any potentially harmful talc or petroleum ingredients often found in commercial products.

Chamomile-Echinacea Gel

Makes about ½ cup

Aloe, chamomile, and echinacea combine to provide gentle relief for your child's rash. Echinacea specifically targets yeast, a common fungus that can exacerbate diaper rash. This gel can maintain its freshness for a duration of 2 weeks when stored in the refrigerator.

Ingredients

1 tablespoon dried chamomile

1 tablespoon chopped dried echinacea root

½ cup water

¼ cup aloe vera gel

Steps

Mix the chamomile and echinacea together in a saucepan with the water. Heat the mixture until it reaches a boiling point, then reduce the heat to a gentle simmer. Continue cooking the mixture until it has been reduced by half, then remove it from the heat and allow it to cool completely.

Wet a piece of cheesecloth and position it over the top of a funnel. Pour the mixture through the funnel into a glass bowl. Press the cheesecloth firmly to ensure all the liquid is fully extracted.

Mix the aloe vera gel with the liquid using a whisk. Put the finished gel into a glass jar that has been sterilized. Ensure that the jar is tightly sealed and stored in the refrigerator.

After each diaper change, delicately apply a thin layer to the affected areas using a cotton cosmetic pad. Make sure the gel is completely absorbed before applying the Comfrey-Thyme Salve and putting on a new diaper. It is important to continue using this gel for at least 3 days after the diaper rash has cleared up.

Precautions: Do not use echinacea if your baby has an autoimmune disorder.

Comfrey-Thyme Salve

Makes about 1 cup

Comfrey is renowned for its remarkable healing properties, while thyme possesses potent antibacterial effects. This high-quality salve also provides a barrier against moisture, helping to promote healing for your baby's sensitive skin. Consider making a double batch and keeping one jar in your diaper bag and another near your home changing area. This salve can be stored for up to one year in a cool, dark place.

Ingredients

1 cup light olive oil

1 ounce dried comfrey

1 ounce dried thyme

1 ounce beeswax

Steps

Mix the olive oil, comfrey, and thyme in a slow cooker. Opt for the lowest heat setting, ensure the slow cooker is covered, and allow the herbs to steep in the oil for a duration of 3 to 5 hours. Turn off the heat and allow the infused oil to cool.

Warm a small amount of water in the base of a double boiler until it begins to simmer.

Reduce the heat to a low setting.

Cover the upper part of the double boiler with a cheesecloth. Combine the infused oil and firmly squeeze the cheesecloth to ensure all the oil is extracted.

Get rid of the cheesecloth and the herbs that have been used.

Mix the beeswax with the infused oil and place the double boiler on the base with caution.

Gently heat over a low flame. After the beeswax has fully melted, cautiously remove the pan from the heat source. Make sure to transfer the salve into clean, dry containers and allow it to cool completely before sealing.

After every diaper change, delicately apply a thin layer to your little one's diaper area using either your fingers or a gauze pad. Start with a small amount of salve and adjust as needed.

Dry Skin

Various factors, including lack of hydration, high indoor air temperature, and long hot showers, can all lead to dry skin. Regular moisturizing can provide great benefits, especially when combined with the use of humidifiers and treatments that include soothing herbs.

Chickweed-Aloe Gel

Makes about ½ cup

Chickweed and aloe vera work together to nourish and hydrate the skin. This gel is designed to absorb quickly and leave no odor behind. When kept in a cool environment, it will remain fresh for a duration of 2 weeks.

Ingredients

½ cup water

¼ cup dried chickweed

¼ cup aloe vera gel

Steps

Mix the water and chickweed in a saucepan. Bring the mixture to a vigorous boil over high heat, then carefully reduce the heat to a gentle simmer. Continue cooking the mixture until it is reduced by half, then remove it from the heat and allow it to cool completely.

Take a piece of cheesecloth and gently place it over the opening of a funnel, making sure it is moistened. Transfer the mixture through the funnel into a top-notch glass bowl. Squeeze the cheesecloth firmly to extract all the liquid from the herbs.

Mix the aloe vera gel and liquid together using a whisk. Transfer the completed gel to a squeeze bottle that is clean and BPA-free. Ensure that it is tightly sealed and stored in the refrigerator.

Spread a thin layer on the affected areas twice daily using your fingertips.

Start with a small amount and modify the quantity for future use depending on the dryness of your skin.

Calendula-Comfrey Body Butter

Makes about 2½ cups

Calendula and comfrey have soothing properties that can help heal irritated skin, while the emollients in this product help to keep your skin moisturized. Feel free to add your preferred essential oils to give it a delightful fragrance. When properly stored, it can maintain its freshness for up to a year.

Ingredients

½ cup cocoa butter

½ cup coconut oil

½ cup jojoba oil

½ cup shea butter

2 ounces dried calendula

2 ounces dried comfrey

Steps

Mix together all the ingredients in a slow cooker. Opt for the lowest heat setting, ensure the slow cooker is covered, and allow the herbs to steep for 3 to 5 hours. Turn off the heat and allow the infused oil to cool.

Cover a large mixing bowl with a piece of cheesecloth in a gentle manner. Combine the infused oil and firmly press the cheesecloth to ensure complete extraction of the oil.

Remove the cheesecloth and discard the herbs that have been used.

Place the bowl in the refrigerator and let the mixture cool for about an hour, or until it begins to solidify.

Whip the body butter for 10 minutes using a hand mixer or immersion blender until it reaches a light and fluffy consistency. After chilling the bowl in the refrigerator for 15 minutes, proceed to cautiously transfer the body butter into clean, dry jars with secure lids.

Use a small amount and apply it to dry skin with your fingers. Feel free to customize the amount to your liking and use it daily to achieve a silky and indulgent skin texture.

Earache

The sensory nerve endings in the eardrum respond to pressure, causing an earache. Try herbal remedies as soon as you start feeling any discomfort. Seek advice from a healthcare professional if the pain becomes more severe or continues. Severe ear infections can spread infection or cause permanent hearing loss.

Blue Vervain Infusion and Poultice

Makes 1 treatment

Blue vervain is renowned for its remarkable pain-relieving properties and its remarkable ability to enhance circulation. This treatment has a two-fold impact. The warm poultice offers a comforting sensation to the ear area externally, while the infusion, when ingested, aids in relieving the throat discomfort commonly associated with an earache. The infusion has a bitter taste, so you may want to consider adding a sweetener to help mask its flavor.

Ingredients

2 teaspoons dried blue vervain

1 cup boiling water

Steps

Place the blue vervain in a tea infuser and gently immerse it in a mug. Pour the boiling water over it.

Let the infusion steep for 10 minutes.

Take out the infuser from the water and let it cool down until it's hot but not too hot to touch. Move the blue vervain to a piece of cheesecloth and neatly fold the cloth into a 4-inch square.

Apply the poultice gently to your ear and enjoy the tea at a leisurely pace. To reactivate the poultice for a second use, simply wrap it in a moist towel and heat it in the microwave for 5 to 10 seconds.

Continue the treatment up to three times per day until your earache subsides.

Garlic-Mullein Infused Oil

Makes 2 tablespoons

Garlic and mullein flowers have powerful antibacterial and anti-inflammatory properties that can effectively alleviate an earache in no time. This oil has a long shelf life of up to a year when stored in a cool, dark place.

Ingredients

2 tablespoons light olive oil

2 teaspoons crushed or finely chopped dried or freeze-dried garlic

2 teaspoons dried mullein flowers

Steps

Heat a small amount of water in the base of a double boiler until it simmers gently.

Reduce the heat to a lower setting.

Mix the olive oil, garlic, and mullein flowers in a glass measuring cup.

Place the measuring cup in the upper part of the double boiler and allow the herbs to infuse in the oil for a period of 3 to 5 hours. Turn off the heat and allow the infused oil to cool.

Put a piece of cheesecloth carefully over a small bowl. Once the infused oil is added, carefully wring and twist the cheesecloth to ensure that every last drop of oil is extracted. Take out the cheesecloth and discard the used herbs.

Place the infused oil into a clean, sterilized bottle with a dropper top and allow it to cool completely before sealing.

Apply 2 to 3 drops into the ear using the dropper top. Place a cotton ball in the ear and leave it in for 15 minutes. Keep up with this routine two or three times a day until the earache improves.

Precautions: Garlic may cause a skin rash in sensitive individuals; discontinue if irritation occurs.

Eczema

Eczema, or atopic dermatitis, features irritated patches of thick, red, scaly skin that often itch intensely. This skin condition tends to appear and disappear, often aligning with seasonal or dietary allergy symptoms.

Calendula-Goldenseal Spray

Makes 1 cup

Calendula and goldenseal provide antiseptic and anti-inflammatory benefits, while witch hazel helps to soothe redness, itching, and scaling. This spray will remain fresh for up to a year if stored in a cool, dark place.

Ingredients

1 ounce dried calendula

1 ounce dried goldenseal root

¼ cup jojoba oil

¾ cup witch hazel

Steps

Mix the calendula, goldenseal, and jojoba oil in a slow cooker. Select the lowest heat setting, cover the slow cooker, and allow the herbs too steep in the oil for 3 to 5 hours. Turn off the heat and allow the infused oil to cool down.

Place a piece of cloth delicately over a bowl. Combine the infused oil and gently press the cheesecloth to ensure all the oil is fully extracted. Get rid of the herbs once you're done with them.

Combine the infused oil and witch hazel in a glass bottle with a spray top, preferably in a dark-colored shade. Please exercise caution when handling.

Use 1 or 2 spritzes on the affected area. Apply the spray in a gentle manner and allow it to fully soak in. Keep up with this routine two or three times per day until the eczema diminishes.

Comfrey Salve

Makes about 1 cup

Comfrey has a reputation for soothing and alleviating irritated, itchy skin. It also helps to smooth rough areas and prevent cracking. Comfrey has the remarkable ability to stimulate cell regeneration, which can speed up the healing process and potentially assist in repairing damage caused by eczema. This salve will remain effective for up to a year when stored in a cool, dark place.

Ingredients

2 ounces dried comfrey

1 cup light olive oil

1 ounce beeswax

20 drops vitamin E oil

Steps

Mix the comfrey and olive oil in a slow cooker. Opt for the lowest heat setting, ensure the slow cooker is covered, and allow the herbs to steep in the oil for a duration of 3 to 5 hours. Turn off the heat and allow the infused oil to cool down.

Warm up a small amount of water in the base of a double boiler until it reaches a gentle simmer.

Reduce the heat to a low setting.

Cover the top of the double boiler with a piece of cheesecloth. Include the infused oil and carefully press the cheesecloth to ensure all the oil is fully extracted.

Get rid of the cheesecloth and herbs once you're done with them.

Mix the beeswax with the infused oil and place the double boiler on the base with caution.

Gently heat over a low flame. After the beeswax has fully melted, cautiously take the pan off the heat source. Once the mixture has cooled slightly, you can easily add the vitamin E oil by whisking it in. Make sure to transfer the salve into clean, dry containers and allow it to cool completely before sealing.

Use a small amount on areas affected by eczema, adjusting the amount as needed. Keep up with this routine two or three times per day until the eczema gradually diminishes.

Fever

Embrace the natural power of fever as your body fights infection. If your fever worsens or persists, try using certain herbs to help reduce it. Be very careful and proactive in seeking medical assistance if your child has a fever. Promptly seek medical attention if an infant under 4 months old has a body temperature of 100.4°F or higher. Seek prompt medical attention for older children with a fever of 104°F or higher.

Feverfew Syrup

Makes about 2 cups

Feverfew is known for its ability to effectively reduce fevers. This syrup is perfect for children as it is gentle and easy to take. Plus, it can stay fresh for up to 6 months when refrigerated.

Ingredients

2 ounces dried feverfew

2 cups water

1 cup honey

Steps

Combine the feverfew and water in a saucepan. Simmer the liquid over low heat, partially covering it with a lid, until it is reduced by half.

Pour the contents of the saucepan into a glass measuring cup, then strain the mixture through a dampened piece of cheesecloth back into the saucepan, squeezing out the liquid from the cheesecloth.

Include the honey and gently heat the mixture on low, stirring continuously until it reaches a temperature of 105°F to 110°F.

Transfer the syrup to a sterilized jar or bottle and keep it in the refrigerator.

Take 1 tablespoon by mouth three times daily until your symptoms improve.

For optimal results, it is recommended that children under the age of 12 take 1 teaspoon three times per day.

Blue Vervain–Raspberry Leaf Tincture

Makes about 2 cups

Blue vervain and raspberry leaf are highly effective in reducing fever in a gentle manner. This tincture will stay fresh for up to 6 years if stored in a cool, dark place.

Ingredients

4 ounces dried blue vervain

4 ounces dried raspberry leaf

2 cups unflavored 80-proof vodka

Steps

Mix the herbs together in a clean pint jar. Make sure to carefully pour the vodka into the jar, ensuring it completely covers the herbs and fills the jar to the top.

Ensure that the jar is tightly secured and vigorously shake it. Store it in a cool, dark cabinet and remember to give it a gentle shake once a week for 6 to 8 weeks. If any of the alcohol evaporates, just add more vodka to fill the jar to the top once again.

Dampen a piece of cheesecloth and gently position it over the top of a funnel. Pour the tincture into a fresh pint jar using the funnel. Get the liquid out of the herbs by applying pressure to the cheesecloth until all the liquid is released. Take out the roots and transfer the finished tincture into dark glass bottles with caution.

Take 10 drops orally two or three times per day. If the taste is too strong for your preference, you can choose to lessen it by diluting it with a glass of water or juice and drinking it.

Flu

The virus that causes the flu frequently mutates and often leads to symptoms resembling those of the common cold. Get a yearly flu shot, especially if you frequently come into contact with sick individuals or belong to a high-risk group. Catch the flu? Use herbs to relieve your symptoms and speed up your recovery.

Catnip-Hyssop Tea

Makes 1 cup

Both catnip and hyssop have anti-inflammatory properties that can help alleviate symptoms such as a sore throat and body ache. Additionally, they can enhance your immune system, helping to combat the flu virus. This tea is incredibly soothing and perfect for enjoying before a nap or bedtime.

Ingredients

1 cup boiling water

1 teaspoon dried catnip

1 teaspoon dried hyssop

Steps

Transfer the hot water into a spacious mug. Include the dried herbs, place a lid on the mug, and let the tea steep for 10 minutes.

Take your time and savor the tea as you enjoy the soothing steam. Can be repeated up to four times daily.

Precautions: Do not use hyssop or catnip during pregnancy. Omit the hyssop if you have epilepsy

Garlic, Echinacea, and Goldenseal Syrup

Makes 2 cups

Garlic, echinacea, and goldenseal are powerful antiviral herbs that can support your body's natural defense against the flu. This syrup has a strong flavor despite the honey; you might find it more enjoyable if you consume it with a teaspoon of lemon juice. When stored in a cool environment, it can maintain its freshness for up to 6 months.

Ingredients

1 ounce dried or freeze-dried garlic, chopped

1 ounce dried echinacea root, chopped

1 ounce dried goldenseal root, chopped

2 cups water

1 cup honey

Steps

Mix the herbs and water in a saucepan. Warm the liquid slowly until it reaches a gentle simmer. Partially cover it with a lid and allow the liquid to reduce by half.

Transfer the contents of the saucepan into a glass measuring cup. Next, filter the mixture back into the saucepan by using a moistened cheesecloth. Continue squeezing the cheesecloth until all the liquid has been extracted.

Add the honey and heat the mixture over low heat, stirring constantly until it reaches a temperature of 105°F to 110°F.

Place the syrup into a sterilized container and store it in the refrigerator to keep it chilled.

Administer 1 tablespoon orally three times a day until your symptoms show signs of improvement.

For best results, it is advised that children below the age of 12 consume 1 teaspoon three times a day.

Precautions: Do not use echinacea if you are allergic to ragweed or have an autoimmune disease.

Gingivitis

Despite consistent brushing, gingivitis can still occur. This dental problem frequently results in gum recession and, over time, can lead to teeth becoming loose. Incorporate flossing into your daily routine and remember to schedule dental cleanings twice a year. Incorporating herbs into your oral care routine can help support the health of your teeth and gums, alongside regular visits to the dentist for professional cleanings.

Calendula-Chamomile Mouth Rinse

Makes 2 cups

Calendula and chamomile work together to soothe inflammation and combat infections. This mouth rinse has a delightful floral flavor and provides relief to sore gums, promoting the healing of damaged tissue. This rinse can stay fresh for up to a week if stored in the refrigerator.

Ingredients

1 ounce dried calendula

1 ounce dried chamomile

4 cups water

Steps

Mix the herbs and water in a saucepan. Gradually warm the liquid until it reaches a gentle simmer. Then, partially cover it with a lid and allow it to reduce by half.

Transfer the contents of the saucepan into a glass measuring cup. Afterward, filter the mixture back into the saucepan by using a piece of cheesecloth that has been moistened. Give the cheesecloth a good squeeze to get rid of any leftover liquid.

Transfer the mouth rinse to a clean jar or bottle and store it in a cool place.

Take 2 tablespoons twice a day until you start feeling better. It is important to remember to spit the rinse into the sink instead of swallowing it. For children under age 12, it is advised to consume 1 tablespoon twice per day.

Goldenseal-Sage Oil Pull

Makes 24 treatments

This recipe combines goldenseal, sage, and coconut oil to create a potent treatment that aids in reducing inflammation and promoting the healing of sore gums. If you are new to oil pulling, it's best to start slowly and gradually increase the duration of your treatment.
This blend will remain fresh for up to 6 months if stored in a cool, dark place.

Ingredients

1 ounce dried goldenseal root, chopped

1 ounce dried sage, crumbled

½ cup coconut oil

Steps

Mix the herbs and coconut oil in a slow cooker. Select the lowest heat setting, cover the slow cooker, and allow the herbs to steep in the oil for 3 to 5 hours. Turn off the heat and allow the infused oil to cool down.

Place a soft piece of cloth over a bowl. Combine the infused oil and firmly press the cheesecloth to ensure complete extraction of the oil. Take out the cheesecloth and discard the used herbs.

Place the infused coconut oil into a clean, dry jar and allow it to cool completely before sealing.

Take 1 teaspoon of the oil pulling solution and allow it to dissolve in your mouth. Carefully maneuver it around and between your teeth, being cautious not to ingest it. Keep the solution in your mouth for up to 15 minutes, making any necessary adjustments to the amount.

After finishing the task, you can properly dispose of the used oil by absorbing it with a paper towel and then throwing it away in the trash. It is advisable to refrain from disposing of oil down the sink, as it can lead to plumbing problems.

Hair Loss

While hair loss is often thought of as a problem primarily affecting men, it's important to note that women can also experience this condition. Thinning hair can be attributed to a range of factors, such as excessive styling, stress, and vitamin imbalances. While herbs may not be the most effective solution for genetic hair loss, they can still be beneficial for promoting hair growth in other situations.

Ginger Scalp Treatment

Makes ½ cup

Ginger enhances blood flow to the scalp, promoting the activation of hair follicles. This treatment will remain fresh for up to 2 months when stored in the refrigerator.

Ingredients

2 ounces fresh gingerroot, chopped

¼ cup sesame oil

Steps

Mix the ginger and sesame oil in a slow cooker. Opt for the lowest heat setting, ensure the slow cooker is covered, and allow the herbs to steep in the oil for a duration of 3 to 5 hours. Turn off the heat and allow the infused oil to cool down.

Place a soft piece of cloth over a bowl. Combine the infused oil and gently press the cheesecloth to ensure all the oil is extracted. Get rid of the ginger once you're done with it.

Pour the sesame oil into a clean, dry bottle or jar and allow it to cool completely before sealing.

Prior to shampooing, it is recommended to apply 1 tablespoon of the product to the scalp. Handle it with care.

Leave the treatment on for 30 minutes, then proceed to wash and condition your hair as you usually do. Ensure that you repeat three to four times per week.

Precautions: Do not use ginger if you take prescription blood thinners, have gallbladder disease, or have a bleeding disorder.

Ginkgo-Rosemary Tonic

Makes about 1 cup

Ginkgo and rosemary, along with witch hazel, work together to enhance circulation in the scalp, providing a boost to your hair follicles. Rosemary enhances the luster and resilience of your hair, contributing to an enhanced appearance and boosted self-confidence. This tonic will remain fresh for up to 6 months when stored in the refrigerator.

Ingredients

½ ounce dried ginkgo biloba

½ ounce dried rosemary leaves

2 tablespoons fractionated coconut oil

1 cup witch hazel

Steps

Combine the herbs and fractionated coconut oil in a slow cooker. Choose the lowest heat setting, cover the slow cooker, and let the herbs steep in the oil for 3 to 5 hours. Disable the heat and let the infused oil cool down.

Place a piece of cheesecloth gently over a bowl. Add the infused oil and squeeze the cheesecloth tightly until all the oil is extracted. Remove the cheesecloth and used herbs.

Mix the witch hazel with the infused oil in a glass bottle with a spray top. Shake gently to ensure thorough blending.

After washing and conditioning your hair, simply apply a light mist of 1 or 2 spritzes to areas where hair loss is a concern, adjusting the amount as necessary.

Gently massage the scalp using your fingertips. Make sure to repeat once or twice per day.

Precautions: Do not use ginkgo biloba if you are taking a monoamine oxidase inhibitor (MAOI) for depression. Ginkgo biloba enhances the effect of blood thinners; talk to your doctor before use. Do not use rosemary if you have epilepsy.

Halitosis

Unpleasant and embarrassing, having bad breath can be quite bothersome. Luckily, it's also quite easy to resolve. Start by making sure you stay adequately hydrated, as a dry mouth can provide a perfect environment for bacteria to thrive. It is important to prioritize oral hygiene by being thorough with brushing and flossing. If herbal remedies do not yield the desired results, it is recommended to seek guidance from a medical professional. Chronic halitosis may indicate an undisclosed health condition.

Peppermint-Sage Mouthwash

Makes about 2 cups

Peppermint and sage work together to keep your breath fresh, while the powerful formula in this mouthwash effectively eliminates germs. When prepared with vodka and stored in a cool, dark place, the rinse can maintain its freshness for a remarkable 6 years.

Ingredients

6 ounces dried peppermint

2 ounces dried sage

2 cups unflavored 80-proof vodka

Steps

Mix the herbs together in a clean pint jar. Make sure to fill the jar all the way to the top with vodka, ensuring that the herbs are completely submerged.

Ensure that the jar is tightly sealed and vigorously shake it. Store it in a cool, dark cabinet and remember to shake it occasionally for 6 to 8 weeks. If any of the alcohol evaporates, just add more vodka to fill the jar.

Take a piece of cheesecloth and gently place it over the opening of a funnel, making sure it is moistened. Pour the tincture into a fresh pint jar using the funnel. Extract the liquid from the herbs. Properly discard the used herbs and transfer the finished tincture into glass bottles of a dark hue.

After brushing your teeth, it's recommended to rinse with 1 tablespoon of mouthwash. It is recommended to perform this task at least twice a day, and if desired, you may choose to do it more frequently.

Ginger-Mint Gunpowder Green Tea

Makes about 30 servings.

When lemon and spearmint are combined with gunpowder green tea, the polyphenols present in the tea act as antioxidants. These antioxidants have the ability to eliminate certain compounds that are linked to issues like bad breath, tooth decay, and even mouth cancer.

Ingredients

2 lemons

1 (4-inch) piece gingerroot

2 bunches spearmint

1 cup gunpowder green tea leaves

1 cup boiling water

Steps

Get the lemons ready by peeling them, getting rid of the pith, and slicing the rinds into thin slivers.

Place the rinds on a metal rack. (The juiced lemons can be saved for another purpose.)

Peel the ginger and slice it into thin pieces. Place them on the rack alongside the lemon rinds.

Remove the leaves from the spearmint stems, being careful to keep the leaves intact. Take off the stems and place the spearmint leaves on the rack with the lemon rinds and gingerroot.

Let the lemon rinds, gingerroot, and spearmint leaves dry naturally at room temperature until they become completely dry and brittle, typically within 24 hours. Make sure to thoroughly remove any remaining moisture. Crush the spearmint leaves into tiny pieces.

Mix together the lemon rinds, ginger, spearmint leaves, and tea leaves in a large bowl. After all the ingredients are thoroughly mixed, you should take extra care when transferring the mixture into a container with a secure seal. Maintain a moderate temperature for a month.

To make the tea, pour the hot water into a large mug. Place 2 teaspoons of the tea mixture into the mug, then cover it and allow the tea to steep for 10 minutes.

Indulge in a soothing cup of tea.

Hangover

It's not uncommon to overindulge, but there's no reason to endure the full consequences in complete discomfort. Discover effective solutions for addressing common symptoms like headache, nausea, and fatigue, while also incorporating natural remedies that support the detoxification process.

Feverfew-Hops Tea

Makes 1 cup

Feverfew can effectively address your headache, while hops have a calming effect to help you relax. This tea has a powerful effect that can assist you in falling asleep, allowing your body to recuperate more quickly.

Ingredients

1 cup boiling water

1 teaspoon dried feverfew

1 teaspoon dried hops

Steps

Transfer the hot water into a spacious mug. Include the dried herbs, place a lid on the mug, and let the tea steep for 10 minutes.

Take your time and savor the tea. Can be repeated up to three times per day.

Milk Thistle Tincture

Makes about 2 cups

Milk thistle is beneficial for the liver as it aids in the detoxification process. This solution may not provide instant relief, but it can help alleviate some strain on your system. When stored in an optimal environment, the product can maintain its freshness for an extended period of time.

Ingredients

8 ounces dried milk thistle

2 cups unflavored 80-proof vodka

Steps

Place the milk thistle in a sanitized pint jar. Fill the jar to the brim with vodka, ensuring that the herbs are completely submerged.

Make sure to secure the jar firmly and give it a good shake. Keep it in a cool, dark cabinet and give it a good shake every week for 6 to 8 weeks. If any of the alcohol evaporates, simply add more vodka to fill the jar to the top once again.

Moisten a piece of cheesecloth and carefully place it over the opening of a funnel. Transfer the tincture through the funnel into a clean, sterilized pint jar. Extract the liquid from the herbs by firmly squeezing the cheesecloth until all the liquid has been released. Dispose of the used herbs and pour the completed tincture into glass bottles with a dark color.

Take 10 drops orally two or three times per day for 7 to 10 days after excessive consumption. If the flavor is too intense for your liking, you have the option to dilute it by mixing it with water or juice before consumption. If you prefer not to consume alcohol, you can incorporate the tincture into a cup of tea prepared with boiling water. The alcohol will evaporate in approximately 5 minutes.

Headache

Headaches can be caused by a variety of factors, including stress, muscle tension, caffeine withdrawal, eyestrain, and high blood pressure. If you frequently or consistently suffer from headaches, it is recommended to seek guidance from a medical expert, as they could be a sign of an underlying health issue.

Blue Vervain–Catnip Tea

Makes 1 cup

Blue vervain and catnip work in harmony to enhance circulation and induce a sense of calm, while also providing relief from tension. This blend is perfect for relieving stress headaches.

Ingredients

1 cup boiling water

1 teaspoon dried blue vervain

1 teaspoon dried catnip

Steps

Transfer the hot water into a spacious mug. Include the dried herbs, place a lid on the mug, and let the tea steep for 10 minutes.

Take your time and savor the tea. Feel free to repeat this up to three times per day.

Skullcap Tincture

Makes about 2 cups

Skullcap is a gentle sedative that can provide relief for nerve pain. If you experience migraines and are unable to use feverfew, skullcap may be a viable alternative to explore.

This tincture offers fast relief. If you would prefer a more convenient option, skullcap is also available in capsule form. When stored in an optimal environment, this tincture can maintain its freshness for an impressive duration of 6 years.

Ingredients

8 ounces skullcap

2 cups unflavored 80-proof vodka

Steps

Place the skullcap in a sanitized pint jar. Fill the jar to the brim with vodka, ensuring that the herbs are completely submerged.

Make sure to securely seal the jar and give it a good shake. Keep it in a cool, dark cabinet and give it a good shake every few days for 6 to 8 weeks. If any of the alcohol evaporates, make sure to replenish it with more vodka until the jar is completely filled again.

Moisten a piece of cheesecloth and carefully place it over the opening of a funnel. Transfer the tincture through the funnel into a clean pint jar. Extract the liquid from the herbs by firmly squeezing the cheesecloth until all the liquid has been released. Dispose of the used herbs and pour the completed tincture into glass bottles of a dark color.

For headache relief, simply take 1 teaspoon orally two or three times per day. If the flavor is too intense for your liking, you have the option to dilute it by mixing it with water or juice before consumption.

Heartburn

The unpleasant sensation caused by heartburn is a frequent symptom of gastroesophageal reflux disease (GERD), a digestive disorder that happens when stomach acid moves into the esophagus. GERD can be caused by a variety of factors, including excessive acid production, obesity, overeating, wearing tight clothing, and other similar factors. If you're expecting, heartburn might be a common occurrence as your growing baby puts added pressure on your stomach.

Using herbs can offer temporary relief for heartburn while you explore the underlying cause.

Fresh Ginger Tea

Makes 1 cup

Ginger enhances blood circulation throughout the body and can expedite recovery from heartburn. The soothing properties of this product help alleviate the irritation in your esophagus caused by stomach acid.

Ingredients

1 cup boiling water

1 tablespoon chopped fresh gingerroot

Steps

Transfer the hot water into a spacious mug. Include the ginger, place a lid on the mug, and let the tea steep for 10 minutes.

Take your time and savor the tea as you enjoy the soothing steam. Use up to four times per day as needed for heartburn relief.

Fennel-Angelica Syrup

Makes 2 cups

Fennel and angelica enhance blood circulation in the digestive system and provide a soothing effect to an irritated esophagus, promoting faster digestion. This syrup has a long shelf life of 6 months when stored in the refrigerator.

Ingredients

1 ounce dried angelica

1 tablespoon fennel seeds

2 cups water

1 cup honey

Steps

Combine the herbs and water in a saucepan. Simmer the liquid gently over low heat, covering it partially with a lid, until it is reduced by half.

Pour the contents of the saucepan into a glass measuring cup. Then, strain the mixture back into the saucepan using a dampened piece of cheesecloth, squeezing out all the liquid.

Incorporate the honey and gently heat the mixture on a low flame, ensuring to stir continuously until the temperature reaches 105°F to 110°F.

Transfer the syrup to a sterilized jar or bottle and keep it in the refrigerator.

Take 1 tablespoon by mouth three times daily until your heartburn symptoms improve.

High Blood Pressure

If left untreated, high blood pressure, also known as hypertension, can greatly increase the risk of early cognitive decline, heart disease, kidney failure, and stroke. Embracing healthy habits such as weight loss, exercise, and meditation can naturally enhance the healing process. If you are unable to lower your blood pressure within 2 months, it is crucial to promptly seek medical attention from a healthcare professional.

Angelica Infusion

Makes 1 quart

Angelica contains compounds that have similar effects to calcium channel blockers, which are commonly prescribed to lower high blood pressure by relaxing and widening blood vessels. This infusion has a slightly bitter taste, but you can easily enhance its flavor by adding a touch of sweetener or juice to your liking. When stored in a cool environment, it will remain fresh for 3 days.

Ingredients

4 teaspoons dried angelica

4 cups boiling water

4 teaspoons fresh lemon juice

Steps

Combine the dried angelica and boiling water in a teapot. Make sure to cover the pot and let the infusion steep for 10 minutes before adding the lemon juice.

Take your time and savor a cup of the infusion. You have the option to refrigerate the remaining portion and enjoy it gradually over the next few days, whether you prefer to reheat it or have it over ice.

Dandelion-Lavender Tincture

Makes about 2 cups

Dandelions are a great natural way to regulate salt levels and reduce blood pressure. The scent and oils of lavender have a calming effect on the nervous system, promoting relaxation and balance.

Ingredients

4 ounces dried dandelion root, finely chopped

4 ounces dried lavender leaves, chopped

2 cups unflavored 80-proof vodka

Steps

Mix the herbs together in a clean pint jar. Fill the jar to the brim with vodka, making sure to completely submerge the herbs.

Ensure that the jar is tightly sealed and give it a thorough shake. Store it in a cool, dark cabinet and remember to give it a gentle shake every few days for 6 to 8 weeks. If any of the alcohol evaporates, be sure to add more vodka until the jar is filled to the brim again.

Place a damp piece of cheesecloth over the opening of a funnel with caution. Pour the tincture into a fresh pint jar using the funnel. Squeeze the cheesecloth firmly to extract all the liquid from the herbs. Properly discard the used herbs and transfer the finished tincture into glass bottles of a dark hue.

Take 10 drops orally two or three times per day. If the taste is too strong for your preference, you can choose to lessen it by blending it with a glass of water or juice before drinking. Continue your dedication to improving your lifestyle and taking proactive measures to support your blood pressure.

Precautions: It is recommended to refrain from using this tincture for longer than 2 months. Overconsumption of dandelions can lead to a notable reduction in blood pressure levels, which may pose potential risks. Consuming lavender in large quantities can lead to side effects such as constipation, headaches, and increased appetite. If you experience any adverse reactions, it is crucial to promptly consult with your doctor for medical guidance.

Indigestion

Experiencing symptoms such as bloating, belching, and discomfort can be signs that something you ate didn't agree with your stomach or that you may have overindulged in a favorite dish. Herbs offer quick relief without the potential side effects that can accompany commercial antacids.

Chamomile-Angelica Tea

Makes 1 cup

Angelica and chamomile have a soothing effect on the muscles in the gastrointestinal tract, promoting better circulation and maintaining a healthy flow. Adding a teaspoon of honey and a squeeze of fresh lemon can enhance the taste of your tea.

Ingredients

1 cup boiling water

1 teaspoon dried angelica

1 teaspoon dried chamomile

Steps

Transfer the hot water into a spacious mug. Include the dried herbs, cover the mug, and let the tea steep for 10 minutes.

Take your time and savor the tea. Repeat up to four times daily.

Ginger Syrup

Makes 2 cups

Ginger has a calming effect on the digestive tract and promotes better blood circulation, which can aid in digestion. For even faster relief, try taking this remedy with a teaspoon of fresh lemon juice. This syrup can be stored in the refrigerator for up to 6 months while maintaining its freshness.

Ingredients

2 ounces fresh gingerroot, chopped

2 cups water

1 cup honey

Steps

Mix the ginger and water in a saucepan. Warm the liquid slowly until it reaches a gentle simmer. Partially cover it with a lid and allow the liquid to reduce by half.

Transfer the contents of the saucepan to a glass measuring cup, and strain the mixture back into the saucepan using a dampened piece of cheesecloth. Give the cheesecloth a good squeeze to get rid of any excess liquid.

Combine the honey and heat the mixture over a low flame, making sure to stir constantly until it reaches a temperature of 105°F to 110°F.

Place the syrup into a sterilized container and store it in the refrigerator.

Take one tablespoon orally three or four times daily until your symptoms show improvement. For children under age 12, it is advised to take 1 teaspoon up to three times per day.

Insect Bites

Mosquitos, chiggers, biting gnats, and fleas are some of the pests that can cause bothersome, itchy bites on your skin. At times, these irritating bites can be quite bothersome, leading to discomfort that can interfere with concentration and a restful night's sleep. Thankfully, there are natural solutions that can offer relief.

Fresh Basil-Mullein Salve

Makes 1 treatment

Basil and mullein offer anti-inflammatory benefits, with basil also containing eugenol, a constituent renowned for its itch-numbing properties. This remedy harnesses the natural properties of honey to effectively bind the herbs to your skin, facilitating faster healing of your bug bites. If you have a significant number of insect bites or if your entire family is affected, you can effortlessly scale up the recipe to ensure there is an ample amount for everyone. When kept in the refrigerator, it stays fresh for about 2 days.

Ingredients

1 tablespoon fresh basil

1 tablespoon fresh mullein

1 tablespoon raw honey

Steps

Combine all the ingredients in a mini food processor. Blend the ingredients until they form a smooth paste.

Using your fingertip or a cotton swab, gently apply a small amount of the blend to each of your insect bites.

Store any remaining salve in a small container with a secure lid and keep it refrigerated for future use. Continue the treatment whenever itching resurfaces.

Peppermint-Plantain Balm

Makes about 5 tablespoons (enough to fill 5 lip balm tubes)

If you frequently encounter buggy environments, you'll appreciate the convenience and user-friendly nature of these tubes of insect bite balm. The peppermint and plantain provide soothing relief and promote faster healing for your skin. Additionally, this balm can be used to keep your lips feeling soft and smooth. This remedy has a long shelf life of up to a year when stored in a cool, dark place.

Ingredients

1 tablespoon dried peppermint

1 tablespoon dried plantain

2 tablespoons jojoba oil

1 tablespoon light olive oil

1 tablespoon cocoa butter

4 teaspoons grated beeswax or beeswax pastilles

3 drops vitamin E oil

20 drops peppermint essential oil (optional)

Steps

Mix the herbs with the jojoba oil, olive oil, and cocoa butter in a slow cooker. Opt for the lowest heat setting, ensure the slow cooker is covered, and allow the herbs to steep in the oil for a duration of 3 to 5 hours. Turn off the heat and allow the infused oil to cool.

Warm a small amount of water in the base of a double boiler until it reaches a gentle simmer.

Reduce the heat to a low setting.

Cover the upper section of the double boiler with a piece of cheesecloth. Once the infused oil is added, carefully squeeze and twist the cheesecloth until every last drop of oil has been extracted. Get rid of the cheesecloth and herbs once you're done with them.

Mix the beeswax with the infused oil and place the double boiler on the base with caution.

Remove the pan from the heat after the wax has melted, and add the vitamin E oil and peppermint essential oil if you prefer. Transfer the mixture into empty lip balm tubes or tins and allow it to cool completely before sealing.

Use a small amount of balm on each insect bite whenever needed to relieve itching.

Laryngitis

When the voice box becomes swollen and inflamed due to infection, irritation, or overuse, laryngitis can occur. If the issue continues, it is recommended to seek medical advice as prolonged hoarseness could be a sign of an underlying condition. Although herbs can offer some relief, it is advisable to seek professional medical attention.

Mullein-Sage Tea

Makes 1 cup

Mullein and sage can provide relief and promote healing for laryngitis symptoms and irritated tissue. This calming solution possesses a potent herbal flavor; you might consider incorporating a teaspoon of lemon juice or honey to enhance its palatability.

Ingredients

1 cup boiling water

1 teaspoon dried mullein

1 teaspoon dried sage

Steps

Transfer the hot water into a spacious mug. Include the dried herbs, cover the mug, and let the tea steep for 10 minutes.

Indulge in a moment of pure relaxation as you savor your favorite tea. Feel free to repeat as often as needed.

Ginger Gargle

Makes 1 cup

This recipe includes ginger, which can help alleviate pain and reduce inflammation in your throat. The addition of honey provides a gentle coating and extra anti-inflammatory properties. If you're interested, you can also use this recipe to make a calming tea.

Ingredients

1 cup boiling water

1 teaspoon minced fresh or dried ginger

1 teaspoon honey

Steps

Transfer the hot water into a spacious mug. Include the ginger and honey, cover the mug, and let the mixture steep for 10 minutes.

Allow the liquid to cool to room temperature or refrigerate it for a cooler experience. Take 1 tablespoon at a time and repeat as necessary to soothe throat irritation. Keep refrigerated for up to 3 days.

Menopause

Menopause is a normal phase in a woman's hormonal cycle, but unfortunately, it can bring about physical discomfort.
In addition to these natural remedies, it can be beneficial to include regular physical activity and a diet that includes non-GMO soy, which is a natural source of plant estrogen..

Fennel-Sage Decoction

Makes 1 cup

This fennel and sage decoction provides estrogenic properties and can be helpful in managing hot flashes when they occur. You have the option to make a larger batch if you prefer, and you can store it in the refrigerator for up to a week for convenience. You may consider adding a sweetener to enhance the flavor, if desired.

Ingredients

2 cups water

1 teaspoon fennel seeds

1 teaspoon sage

Steps

Combine all the ingredients in a saucepan and bring to a boil over high heat.

Lower the heat and let the mixture simmer until the liquid is reduced by half.

Allow the decoction to cool for a few minutes. Enjoy a leisurely drink of the full quantity.

Black Cohosh Tincture

Makes about 2 cups

Black cohosh contains isoflavones that mimic the hormonal activity commonly found in females. It can be beneficial in addressing the symptoms often associated with menopause, including mild depression, vaginal dryness, and hot flashes. This tincture can remain fresh for up to 6 years if stored in a cool, dark place.

Ingredients

8 ounces black cohosh, finely chopped

2 cups unflavored 80-proof vodka

Steps

Place the black cohosh in a sterilized pint jar. Fill the jar to the brim with vodka, ensuring that the herbs are fully submerged.

Make sure to seal the jar securely and give it a good shake. Keep it in a cool, dark cabinet and give it a gentle shake a few times each week for 6 to 8 weeks. If any of the alcohol evaporates, make sure to replenish it with more vodka until the jar is completely filled again.

Moisten a piece of cheesecloth and place it gently over the opening of a funnel. Transfer the tincture through the funnel into a clean pint jar. Extract the liquid from the herbs by firmly squeezing the cheesecloth until all the liquid has been released. Dispose of the used herbs and carefully pour the completed tincture into glass bottles with a dark hue.

Take half a teaspoon by mouth once daily. If the flavor is too intense for your liking, you have the option to dilute the tincture by mixing it into a glass of water or juice before consumption.

Mental Wellness

Challenging professions, packed agendas, and draining experiences can leave you feeling anxious, downcast, and low on energy. Using herbs can have a significant impact, but it's important to prioritize safety and always consult your doctor before making any changes to your prescription medication.

St. John's Wort Tea

Makes 1 cup

While this remedy is simple and straightforward, it is highly effective for managing anxiety and minor depression. If tea isn't your cup of tea, consider trying a top-notch St. John's wort supplement and follow the recommended dosage.

Ingredients

1 cup boiling water

1 teaspoon dried St. John's wort

Steps

Pour the boiling water into a large mug. Add the St. John's wort, cover the mug, and allow the tea too steep for 10 minutes.

Relax and drink the tea slowly while inhaling the steam. Repeat up to two times per day.

Chamomile-Passionflower Decoction

Makes 1 cup

Chamomile and passionflower are known for their calming properties, helping to promote relaxation and alleviate anxiety.

This blend is incredibly calming and can assist in achieving a more restful sleep, particularly during times of worry-induced insomnia. Feel free to enhance the flavor if you prefer.

Ingredients

2 cups water

1 teaspoon dried chamomile

1 teaspoon dried passionflower

Steps

Combine all the ingredients in a saucepan and bring to a boil over high heat.

Lower the heat and let the mixture simmer until the liquid is reduced by half.

Allow the decoction to cool for 5 to 10 minutes. Enjoy a leisurely drink of the full quantity.

Precautions: Avoid chamomile if you have allergies to plants in the ragweed family or if you are on prescription blood thinners. Avoid using passionflower if you are pregnant or if you have baldness or prostate problems.

Muscle Cramps

Tight muscles can cause discomfort and muscle contractions, which can affect your ability to move freely and even disturb your sleep.

Utilizing herbs can offer respite from muscle tension and support the body's natural healing process. If you often experience cramps, it is recommended to seek medical advice, as they could be a sign of an underlying medical condition.

Rosemary Liniment

Makes ½ cup

Rosemary has the ability to enhance circulation and contains components that can alleviate discomfort. Enhance the potency of this straightforward solution by incorporating rosemary essential oil. When stored in the refrigerator, the product will remain fresh for a remarkable 7 years.

Ingredients

2 tablespoons rosemary tincture

⅓ Cup unflavored 80-proof vodka

20 drops rosemary essential oil (optional)

Steps

In a dark-colored glass bottle, combine the ingredients by shaking gently.

With a cotton cosmetic pad, apply 5 to 10 drops to the cramped area. Use a little more or less as needed.

Repeat hourly while having cramps or muscle spasms.

Ginger Salve

Makes about 1 cup

Ginger enhances blood circulation and provides a warming sensation that deeply penetrates the skin.

Its exceptional anti-inflammatory and pain-relieving properties make it an excellent choice for addressing muscle cramps.

Ingredients

2 ounces dry or freeze-dried gingerroot, chopped

1 cup light olive oil

1 ounce beeswax

Steps

Mix the ginger and olive oil in a slow cooker. Select the lowest heat setting, cover the slow cooker, and allow the ginger to steep in the oil for 3 to 5 hours. Turn off the heat and allow the infused oil to cool.

Heat a small amount of water until it simmers gently in the base of a double boiler.

Reduce the heat to a lower setting.

Cover the top of the double boiler with a cheesecloth. After adding the infused oil, carefully squeeze and twist the cheesecloth until every last drop of oil is extracted.

Get rid of the cheesecloth and herbs once you're done with them.

Mix the beeswax with the infused oil and place the double boiler on the base with caution.

Gently heat over a low flame. After the beeswax has fully melted, cautiously remove the pan from the heat source. Make sure to transfer the salve into clean, dry containers and allow it to cool completely before sealing.

Delicately apply a small amount to the cramped area using your fingertips.

Modify the quantity as required and repeat as necessary in case of cramping.

Precautions: Do not use ginger if you take prescription blood thinners, have gallbladder disease, or have a bleeding disorder.

Oily Skin

Excessive sebum production can result in oily skin, as it plays a role in moisturizing and waterproofing the skin. Intensive treatments can sometimes lead to excessive dryness of the skin, which may inadvertently stimulate more sebum production and make the issue worse instead of better. Embrace a gentle approach to caring for your oily skin, and finding balance will become much easier.

Rosemary Toner

Makes about 1 cup

Rosemary is a gentle astringent that helps balance skin. The witch hazel that serves as the base for this toner refreshes your skin without drying it out. This toner stays fresh for up to 6 months when stored in the refrigerator.

Ingredients

1 cup witch hazel

2 tablespoons rosemary tincture

Steps

Mix the ingredients by softly shaking them in a bottle with a dark hue.

Apply a small amount to your face using a cotton cosmetic pad. Modify the quantity as needed.

Use this product twice a day or whenever you desire to refresh your skin.

Peppermint Scrub

Makes 1 cup

Peppermint provides a soothing and refreshing sensation to the skin, leaving it clean and revitalized. This recipe contains gentle ingredients and can be used on a daily basis, if desired. This scrub can remain fresh for up to 2 months when stored in a cool, dry place.

Ingredients

1 cup dried peppermint leaves, packed

¾ cup baking soda

Steps

Combine the peppermint leaves and baking soda in a food processor or blender. Continue processing until a fine powder is achieved.

Move the mixture to a fresh container that has a secure lid.

Moisten your face and apply a small amount of the scrub to gently massage your skin, using gentle pressure and circular motions. Remember to rinse thoroughly after you have covered all areas. Make sure to repeat once or twice per day.

Premenstrual Syndrome (PMS)

Irritability, mood swings, bloating, and headaches are commonly reported symptoms of PMS. While many women experience mental and physical discomfort before their monthly period, it can be quite challenging. These remedies have been proven to be highly effective in relieving the symptoms.

Dandelion-Ginger Tea

Makes 1 cup

Dandelion helps alleviate bloating that can occur during PMS, while ginger provides relief for cramps and uplifts your mood. If you enjoy the flavor of this tea and wish to indulge in it more often, preparing a generous amount is a simple task. Store it in a pitcher in the refrigerator, and it will remain fresh for up to a week.

Ingredients

1 cup boiling water

1 teaspoon chopped dandelion root

1 teaspoon chopped gingerroot

Steps

Transfer the hot water into a spacious mug. Include the roots, place a lid on the mug, and let the tea steep for 10 minutes.

Take your time and savor the tea as you enjoy the soothing steam. Can be repeated up to four times per day.

Precautions: Avoid using ginger if you are currently taking prescription blood thinners, have gallbladder disease, or suffer from a bleeding disorder.

Black Cohosh Syrup

Makes about 2 cups

Black cohosh can assist in regulating hormonal activity, providing some relief from PMS symptoms. This syrup has a slightly bitter taste and is a convenient substitute for tea. It can be stored in the refrigerator for up to 6 months.

Ingredients

2 ounces black cohosh

2 cups water

1 cup honey

Steps

Mix the black cohosh and water in a saucepan. Gently heat the liquid, partially covering it with a lid, until it is reduced by half.

Transfer the contents of the saucepan into a glass measuring cup, and strain the mixture back into the saucepan using a piece of cheesecloth that has been dampened. Continue squeezing the cheesecloth until all the liquid has been extracted.

Add the honey and heat the mixture over low heat, stirring constantly until it reaches a temperature of 105°F to 110°F.

Place the syrup into a sterilized jar or bottle and store it in the refrigerator.

Take 1 tablespoon orally three times per day when experiencing PMS symptoms.

Ringworm

Despite its name, ringworm is not caused by a parasite. Actually, it's a fungal infection that appears as red, circular patches with raised edges that resemble blisters. Ringworm is a contagious condition that causes intense itching and can easily spread between individuals, including pets. It is crucial to prioritize hygiene when dealing with this condition, making sure to keep the affected area clean and dry while using antifungal herbs.

Fresh Garlic Compress

Makes 1 compress

Garlic is an effective antifungal agent that efficiently combats ringworm. If you happen to experience an itching and tingling sensation in a specific area without any visible rash, one possible solution is to apply fresh garlic to that spot. This may help prevent the rash from developing.

Ingredients

1 cup steaming-hot water (not boiling)

1 garlic clove, cut in half

Steps

Immerse a gentle cloth in the warm water.

Mash or blend half of the garlic clove and spread the paste onto the area. Place the cloth over it and secure it with a bandage to keep the treatment in place.

If you're in a hurry, place half of the garlic clove over the ringworm rash with the cut side facing down. Place the cloth over it and secure it with a bandage.

Keep the compress on for 10 to 15 minutes, then remove the garlic.

It is recommended to use a fresh piece of garlic for each affected area of ringworm.

Continue the treatment two or three times per day until the ringworm is completely eliminated.

Precautions: Garlic can cause skin irritation in sensitive individuals. Discontinue use if this occurs.

Goldenseal Balm

Makes ½ cup

Goldenseal is a powerful antifungal agent that can provide relief from the itching caused by ringworm. It also has anti-inflammatory properties that can help reduce inflammation. This recipe contains coconut oil, which has antifungal properties and can promote faster healing of the skin. If you happen to have tea tree essential oil available, incorporating it into this recipe will enhance the potency of the balm.

Ingredients

2 ounces dried goldenseal root

¼ cup coconut oil

½ ounce beeswax

20 drops tea tree essential oil (optional)

Steps

Mix the goldenseal and coconut oil in a slow cooker. Opt for the lowest heat setting, ensure the slow cooker is covered, and allow the herbs to steep in the oil for a duration of 3 to 5 hours. Turn off the heat and allow the infused oil to cool down.

Heat a small amount of water until it reaches a gentle simmer in the base of a double boiler.

Reduce the heat to a lower setting.

Cover the upper part of the double boiler with a piece of cheesecloth. Combine the infused oil and gently press the cheesecloth to ensure all the oil is extracted.

Get rid of the herbs after use.

Mix the beeswax with the infused oil and place the double boiler on the base with caution.

Gently heat over a low flame. After the beeswax has completely melted, gently remove the pan from the heat source. If you decide to incorporate it, consider including the tea tree essential oil. Make sure to transfer the salve into clean, dry containers and allow it to cool completely before sealing.

Apply a small amount of the balm to the affected areas where ringworm is a concern using a cotton cosmetic pad or gauze pad. Make sure to apply the product three or four times a day, and don't forget to apply it again before going to bed. It is important to continue the treatment until the ringworm has completely cleared.

Sore Muscles

Usually caused by overexertion or prolonged periods of inactivity, sore muscles need time to heal. Utilizing herbal remedies can offer relief and encourage a sense of calm, while giving yourself the opportunity to rest for a day or two can expedite the healing process.

Ginger-Fennel Massage Oil

Makes 1 cup

Fennel and ginger provide a delightful, comforting sensation that eases and calms tense, achy muscles. This treatment will remain fresh for up to 6 months when stored in a cool, dark place.

Ingredients

1 tablespoon crushed fennel seeds

2 ounces dried gingerroot, chopped

1 cup light olive oil

Steps

Mix together the fennel, ginger, and olive oil in a slow cooker. Opt for the lowest heat setting, ensure the slow cooker is covered, and allow the herbs to steep in the oil for a duration of 3 to 5 hours. Turn off the heat and allow the infused oil to cool down.

Place a soft piece of cloth over a bowl. Squeeze the cheesecloth tightly to ensure all the oil has been extracted. Take out the cheesecloth and discard the used herbs.

Transfer the oil to a container with a dark color and a tightly fitting lid.

Apply a small amount of oil to the desired areas using your fingertips, adjusting the quantity as needed. Experience a massage with a hint of vigor. Use as often as needed to provide pain relief without relying on medication.

Peppermint–St. John's Wort Salve

Makes about 1 cup

Peppermint and St. John's wort offer effective pain relief and promote muscle relaxation. Take caution when using this remedy once it's complete, as the vibrant hue of the St. John's wort may leave stains on clothing. When properly stored, this salve can maintain its freshness for up to a year.

Ingredients

1 cup light olive oil

2 ounces St. John's wort

1 ounce dried peppermint

1 ounce beeswax

Steps

Mix the olive oil, St. John's wort, and peppermint in a slow cooker.

Select the lowest heat setting, cover the slow cooker, and allow the herbs to steep in the oil for 3 to 5 hours. Turn off the heat and allow the infused oil to cool.

Warm a small amount of water in the base of a double boiler until it reaches a gentle simmer.

Reduce the heat to a gentle simmer.

Cover the upper section of the double boiler with a piece of cheesecloth. After adding the infused oil, gently squeeze and twist the cheesecloth until every last drop of oil has been extracted. Get rid of the cheesecloth and herbs once you're done with them.

Mix the beeswax with the infused oil and place the double boiler on the base with caution.

Gently heat over a low flame. After the beeswax has fully melted, cautiously remove the mixture from the heat source. Make sure to transfer the salve into clean, dry containers and allow it to cool completely before sealing.

Apply a small amount of the salve to the affected area using your fingertips, adjusting the quantity as needed. Feel free to repeat as many times as needed to find relief from discomfort.

Sore Throat

No matter what may be causing your sore throat, the discomfort can be quite unpleasant and leave you feeling miserable. Although herbal remedies can be effective, antibiotics may be necessary in the case of a bacterial infection. If you think you might have strep throat, it's crucial to quickly make an appointment with a healthcare professional.

Peppermint Tea with Comfrey and Sage

Makes 1 cup

Peppermint, comfrey, and sage are known for their soothing properties that can help alleviate the discomfort of a sore throat. The comforting warmth of the tea also offers extra relief by reducing inflammation. If you feel that the taste of this tea is too strong for your liking, you can add honey and lemon to adjust the flavor to your preference.

Ingredients

1 cup boiling water

1 teaspoon dried peppermint

1 teaspoon dried comfrey

1 teaspoon dried sage

Steps

Transfer the hot water into a spacious mug. Include the dried herbs, place a lid on the mug, and let the tea steep for 10 minutes.

Take a deep breath and enjoy the soothing tea. Use as directed, up to four times per day as necessary.

Agrimony-Licorice Gargle

Makes 1 cup

Agrimony, licorice, and honey offer a comforting solution for pain relief. If you prefer, you have the option to enjoy this gargle as a tea. If you prefer a refreshing experience, you can refrigerate it before using.

Ingredients

1 cup boiling water

1 tablespoon agrimony

1 teaspoon chopped licorice root

1 teaspoon honey

Steps

Transfer the hot water into a spacious mug. Include the herbs and honey, place a lid on the mug, and let the mixture steep for 10 minutes.

Allow the liquid to cool to room temperature. Take 1 tablespoon at a time and repeat as necessary to alleviate throat discomfort.

Sunburn

While it is important to avoid sunburn, even those who take precautions may still end up getting burned. If you're having trouble sleeping because of discomfort, you might consider adding a herbal sedative to the topical remedies mentioned in this guide. If you're experiencing a severe sunburn, with blisters, intense pain, or any signs of infection, it's crucial to seek medical attention.

Comfrey Spray

Makes about 1 cup

This fast-acting comfrey spray provides rapid relief for sunburns, thanks to the soothing properties of the comfrey tincture and witch hazel. When stored in a cool environment, it will remain fresh for up to a year.

Ingredients

1 cup witch hazel

2 tablespoons comfrey tincture

Steps

Mix the witch hazel and comfrey tincture in a glass bottle with a spray top. Gently shake to blend thoroughly.

Apply 1 or 2 spritzes to each sunburned area, adjusting the amount as necessary.

Make sure to let the spray dry completely before getting dressed, and opt for comfortable, lightweight clothing.

Repeat three or four times daily until your sunburn heals.

Hyssop-Infused Aloe Vera Gel

Makes about ½ cup

Hyssop and aloe vera gel are effective in soothing sunburns and aiding in the healing process. If you prefer not to go through the process of making a hyssop decoction and happen to have hyssop tincture available, you can substitute 1 tablespoon of it for the infusion. This gel can remain fresh for up to 2 weeks when stored in the refrigerator.

Ingredients

2 tablespoons dried hyssop

½ cup water

¼ cup aloe vera gel

Steps

Mix the hyssop and water in a saucepan. Heat the mixture until it reaches a rapid boil, then reduce the heat to a gentle simmer. Continue cooking the mixture until it is reduced by half, then remove it from the heat and allow it to cool completely.

Place a damp cheesecloth over the opening of a funnel. Pour the mixture through the funnel into a glass bowl. Squeeze the cheesecloth firmly to extract all the liquid from the herbs.

Mix the aloe vera gel and liquid together using a whisk. Put the finished gel into a clean glass jar. Ensure that the jar is tightly sealed and stored in the refrigerator.

Apply a thin layer to the affected areas three or four times per day using a cotton cosmetic pad or your fingertips..

Weight Loss

Obesity is a long-term health issue that extends beyond superficial concerns. It can worsen other illnesses while causing discomfort in your own skin. It's definitely true that maintaining a healthy, whole-foods diet and incorporating regular exercise are essential for achieving and sustaining weight loss. It's important to mention that integrating herbs into your daily routine can aid in the transition to a healthier lifestyle and promote a more efficient metabolism.

Dieter's Tea Blend with Chickweed, Dandelion, and Fennel

Makes 1 cup

Chickweed, dandelion, and fennel can aid in weight loss by eliminating toxins and reducing bloating and water retention. Fennel can assist in reducing your appetite, making it somewhat more manageable to resist cravings. This tea blend will remain fresh for up to 2 months when stored in a cool, dry place. If you prefer, you have the option to enhance the flavor of your hot tea with a touch of lemon juice.

Ingredients

3 ounces dried chickweed

3 ounces dried dandelion root, chopped

3 ounces fennel seeds, crushed

1 cup boiling water

Steps

Mix the chickweed, dandelion root, and fennel together in a spacious container that has a secure lid.

Pour two teaspoons of the tea mixture into a large mug. Just pour in the boiling water, cover the mug, and allow the herbs to steep for 10 minutes.

Savor a soothing cup of tea. Enjoy two or three cups daily to aid your weight loss efforts.

Ginseng Tincture

Makes about 2 cups

Ginseng offers numerous benefits such as improved circulation, enhanced mood, and nutritional support during weight loss. This is an excellent source of vitamin B12, which is essential for the production of red blood cells and converting food into energy. This tincture is an excellent overall tonic that will maintain its freshness for up to 6 years when stored in a cool, dry place.

Ingredients

8 ounces Panax ginseng or American ginseng, finely chopped

2 cups unflavored 80-proof vodka

Steps

Put the ginseng in a sterilized pint jar. Add the vodka, filling the jar to the very top and covering the herbs completely.

Cap the jar tightly and shake it up. Store it in a cool, dark cabinet and shake it several times per week for 6 to 8 weeks. If any of the alcohol evaporates, add more vodka so that the jar is again full to the top.

Dampen a piece of cheesecloth and drape it over the mouth of a funnel. Pour the tincture through the funnel into another sterilized pint jar. Squeeze the liquid from the herbs, wringing the cheesecloth until no more liquid comes out. Discard the spent herbs and transfer the finished tincture to dark-colored glass bottles.

Take ½ teaspoon orally each morning for 1 month, and then take 2 weeks off from the remedy. Repeat this cycle as many times as you like.

Section Two

Key Herbs to Discover

Explore a diverse selection of herbal medicine staples, including agrimony and witch hazel. This list omits many commonly available herbs, leaving numerous safe and beneficial ones to explore. These choices remain extremely user-friendly. You can purchase all of them in their complete form, and various convenient options are available, including capsules, salves, tablets, teas, tinctures, and more.

Agrimony

Agrimonia eupatoria, Agrimonia gryposepala

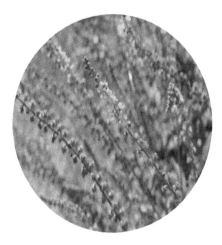

In previous times, agrimony was commonly employed to treat coughs, diarrhea, skin problems, and sore throats. This herb is widely known and has a delightful fragrance that might remind you of the aroma of apricots. It is a wonderful addition to herbal teas, especially when you're not feeling well with a cold or the flu.

Parts Used: Leaves and flowers

Precautions: Can aggravate constipation

Identifying/Growing: Agrimony, a plant belonging to the rose family, is also referred to as the cocklebur or sticklewort. The stem of this plant is covered in soft down, instead of prickly thorns. The branches are covered in sharp, dark green leaves, which later produce clusters of small, vibrant yellow flowers that leave behind prickly burrs after they wither. The plant generally reaches a height of 2 feet on average, although there are instances where it can grow up to 4 feet.

While agrimony is a plant that can be found in fields and woodlands across Europe and North America, it is relatively simple to cultivate. It flourishes in sunny conditions and thrives with consistent watering. Ensuring the soil's moisture levels and proper drainage is crucial.

You are welcome to collect the leaves at any time during the season, and just trim the flowers once they begin to blossom.

Aloe

Aloe vera, Aloe barbadensis, Aloe ferox

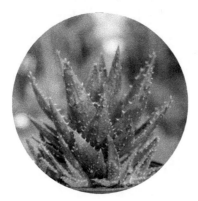

Contrary to its cactus-like appearance, aloe is actually a member of the lily family. The gel found in the thick, spiky leaves possesses remarkable healing properties and can effectively alleviate burns, cuts, and scrapes. Although fresh aloe is undoubtedly beneficial to have on hand, the bottled version is equally potent and offers added convenience.

Parts Used: Gel and juice from inner leaves

Precautions: Aloe juice is a strong laxative. It should not be taken internally during pregnancy or while breastfeeding.

Identifying/Growing: There are over 250 species of aloe that can be found all around the world. Many species have their origins in Africa and display stunning gray-green leaf patterns. The plants also have long, slim stems that produce beautiful yellow, tube-shaped flowers. This plant is rarely found in its natural habitat, unless you live in a tropical region. However, it is quite easy to grow as an indoor plant.

When planting your aloe, it's important to select a container that provides ample space and use soil that drains well. Give it slow-release pellets or a 10-40-10 fertilizer, and ensure consistent watering. It is important to allow the soil to fully dry between waterings, particularly during the winter months when it enters its dormant phase. If you live in a colder area with hot summers, feel free to move your aloe vera plants outdoors when there is no chance of freezing temperatures.

Angelica

Angelica archangelica

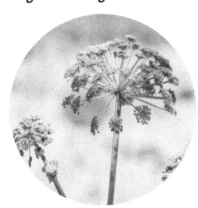

Angelica has a rich history of being utilized as a natural remedy to assist in the induction of labor in instances of delayed childbirth. This herb is incredibly effective at alleviating the discomfort of painful menstruation and cramps. In addition, its ability to relieve congestion and indigestion makes it a valuable choice for meeting the needs of the whole family.

Parts Used: Root, leaves, stems, and fruit

Precautions: Angelica has the ability to enhance blood circulation in the pelvic area and uterus, potentially leading to the initiation of menstruation. It is not recommended for use during pregnancy. This product has elevated levels of coumarin, an organic compound known for its pleasant fragrance and ability to thin the blood. It is important to note that this may potentially interact negatively with anticoagulant medications.

Identifying/Growing: Angelica can be found growing freely in fields and meadows across temperate zones worldwide, especially near streams and rivers. It thrives in partially shaded areas, reaching a height of 3 to 6 feet. A delightful fragrance fills the air as clusters of small, creamy yellow or greenish flowers bloom in late June to July.

Angelica can thrive in a variety of lighting conditions, ranging from partial shade to full sun. Moist, well-drained soil is recommended, along with being close to a water feature. Ensure proper spacing between your plants after germination, allowing them enough room to grow. Only harvest your plants once they have reached full maturity.

Angelica is a biennial plant. By planting it consecutively each year, you can guarantee a yearly harvest.

Arnica

Arnica Montana

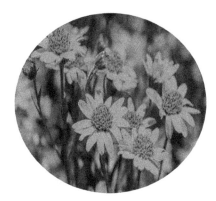

Arnica is an impressive alpine herb known for its exceptional anti-inflammatory properties, which have gained recognition beyond the field of herbal medicine. While arnica creams and oils may be convenient, it is possible to find the whole herb online with ease.

Parts Used: Flowers

Precautions: Do not use in open or bleeding wounds. Long-term use can cause skin irritation.

Identifying/Growing: This fragrant herb, also referred to as mountain arnica, thrives in alpine meadows. The plant features aromatic serrated leaves and bright yellow to orange flowers, similar to daisies, on tall stems that usually grow to be 1 to 2 feet tall. Arnica flourishes in sunny conditions, although it can also handle a bit of shade. If you decide to grow this herb, it does require a certain amount of patience since the seeds can take anywhere from 1 month to 2 years to germinate. You have two choices: you can either sow the seeds outside in late summer or hope for the best, or you can sow them in large pots indoors. They will start growing when the temperature is around 55°F. Once the arnica begins to grow, it will flourish and spread through its roots and by self-seeding. By pruning the plants after they have bloomed, you may be able to experience another beautiful display of flowers. Ensure the well-being of your arnica by regularly dividing the plants at the roots every 3 years, either in the spring or autumn.

Basil

Ocimum basilicum

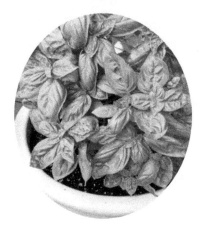

Many people are familiar with the way basil can enhance the flavor of food, as well as its distinct sweet aroma. It is important to mention that there are various types of basil, each possessing distinct antibacterial properties and the ability to provide relief to the stomach. Fresh basil can also be used to soothe insect bites.

Parts Used: Leaves

Precautions: Do not use during pregnancy.

Identifying/Growing: Basil is typically available in the produce department of your local supermarket, although it is not commonly found growing wild. Given its potency and ease of cultivation, fresh basil is a herb worth considering for even the least experienced gardeners. Basil flourishes in the garden or grows just as contentedly in a pot on a sunlit windowsill. It thrives in bright conditions and flourishes in direct sunlight. Regular watering is necessary to maintain the soil's moisture level. By selectively picking the top leaves, you can promote healthy growth and discourage the plant from producing seeds.

Black cohosh

Cimicifuga racemosa

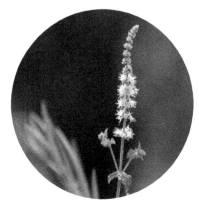

Black cohosh contains isoflavones that have properties resembling estrogen. Black cohosh can be a beneficial choice for addressing symptoms commonly associated with menopause, including vaginal dryness, hot flashes, and mild depression. In addition, it offers benefits that help reduce inflammation and relieve pain. As a highly effective cold and flu remedy, it effectively soothes coughs and provides relief from discomfort.

Parts Used: Root

Precautions: Do not use during pregnancy or breastfeeding. Black cohosh causes gastric discomfort in some individuals; stop using it if this occurs.

Identifying/Growing: Black cohosh is native to the eastern half of North America and tends to thrive in the outskirts of fields and open woodlands. The plant has oval-shaped leaves, tall erect stems that can reach a height of 3 feet or more, and delicate white flowers on slender spikes. Its name is derived from the dark color of its rootstock.

For optimal growth, it is recommended to plant black cohosh seeds in indoor containers during the fall season. It is important to provide them with a warm and dry environment, ideally with ample sunlight exposure. Once the plants start growing, make sure to water them on a weekly basis and keep them indoors until the risk of frost has passed. Consider relocating your black cohosh to a spot that enjoys the gentle touch of morning sunlight, while also providing a comforting shade in the afternoon. Make sure to fertilize the area with well-rotted compost before transplanting and continue this practice each spring. Make sure to water the plants regularly, especially during dry weather. If you see them starting to wilt, increase the frequency of watering.

Blue vervain

Verbena hastata, Verbena officinalis

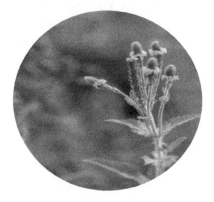

Blue vervain has a reputation for its calming effects on the nervous system and its ability to provide relief from pain. Using poultices can provide relief for conditions like rheumatism, joint pain, and neuralgia. Tea leaves have been known to offer relief for headaches, bladder discomfort, and sore throats. Next time you're dealing with chest congestion or bronchitis, it might be worth considering trying blue vervain tea. It is well-known for its expectorant properties.

Parts Used: Leaves

Precautions: Do not use during pregnancy.

Identifying/Growing: Blue vervain is commonly found growing in meadows, waste places, and along roadsides across North America and Europe. The plant features lance-shaped leaves with rough, toothy edges that are arranged on stems averaging 3 to 7 feet in height. At the top of the plant, slender spikes give rise to beautiful purplish blue flowers.

This delightful herb is a breeze to cultivate. For successful germination of blue vervain, it is important to provide adequate light. To achieve this, sow the seeds and water them without covering them with soil. Remember to keep the seeds adequately watered until they begin to sprout. For more potent solutions, select the herbs prior to their blooming and promptly dry them. If you want a consistent supply year after year, you can let some of your blue vervain flower and go to seed. This way, it will self-seed and return every spring.

Catnip

Nepeta cataria

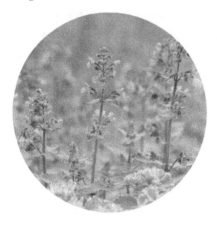

Most people are familiar with catnip, a popular treat for our beloved cats. Although this herb can bring out a cat's playful side, it tends to have the opposite effect on most people. It promotes a state of deep relaxation without any of the negative side effects typically associated with pharmaceutical sedatives.

Parts Used: Leaves and flowering tops

Precautions: Do not use during pregnancy.

Identifying/Growing: Wild catnip is commonly found growing alongside roads. The plant's leaves emit a pleasant minty scent and boast a beautiful greyish-green color with a velvety texture. The upper part of the plant is graced with exquisite white flowers, delicately marked with lavender-colored spots.

Catnip is a delightful addition to any garden. Just like other members of the mint family, it's incredibly easy to grow and has a tendency to spread if not controlled. Start the seeds indoors during the spring season. After the danger of frost has subsided, you can safely move the young seedlings to a spot that receives ample sunlight and has good drainage. Keep your catnip plants safe by using a chicken wire lid to protect them from curious felines. Experience the abundant harvest of leaves and flowers, season after season, year after year.

Chamomile

Matricaria recutita

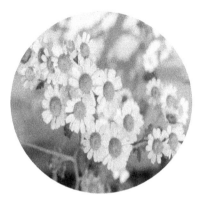

Chamomile possesses gentle yet powerful qualities that provide antibacterial and anti-inflammatory benefits. The calming effect of this ingredient is highly valued in tea blends that promote relaxation and restful sleep. In addition, the antispasmodic properties of this product make it an excellent option for alleviating tension and providing relief for sore muscles. Next time you're feeling overwhelmed, achy, or struggling to get some rest, why not consider giving chamomile a try?

Parts Used: Flowers

Precautions: Chamomile has significant levels of coumarin and may have negative interactions with blood thinners. It may also pose difficulties for individuals with ragweed allergies.

Identifying/Growing: Chamomile is originally from Europe, but it can thrive in various locations with minimal effort. The flowers of this plant are small and daisy-like, with white petals and raised yellow centers. The leaves have a delicate and feathery appearance. It's incredibly simple to cultivate from seed, creating a stunning border in the garden that effortlessly renews itself annually. Harvest the flowers when they are at their peak, and anticipate being able to enjoy two separate cuttings every summer.

Chickweed

Stellaria media

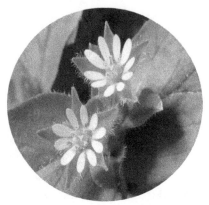

Chickweed is a commonly found wild herb that has a wide distribution across different regions of the globe. Fresh chickweed can be used to make soothing poultices that help with rashes, irritated skin, and minor burns. In addition, the juice can help alleviate itching. Aside from its healing properties, chickweed brings a delightful flavor to fresh spring salads.

Parts Used: Leaves and flowers

Precautions: Consuming large amounts of chickweed may have a laxative effect. Take caution when foraging in locations where chemicals have been used.

Identifying/Growing: Chickweed can be commonly found in lawns, wooded areas, and meadows. This hardy plant flourishes in a range of climates all year round, temporarily retreating during freezing temperatures but quickly reemerging at the first hint of warmth. The plant features elegant white flowers and oval leaves that emerge from slender stems measuring approximately 4 to 6 inches long.

Many people struggle to get rid of chickweed in their lawns, often without much luck.

To ensure optimal growth, create an ideal environment by carefully tending to the soil, ensuring it is adequately hydrated, and spacing the seeds at a distance of approximately ½ inch from each other. Spread a thin layer of topsoil over the area, gently dampen it, and let the plants settle in without any disturbances. Your chickweed will effortlessly spread and flourish without any need for maintenance.

Comfrey

Symphytum officinale

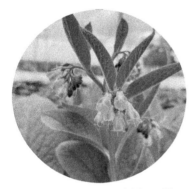

The Latin name of comfrey is derived from the Greek word sympho, which signifies the process of promoting growth and unity. This is commonly used to speed up the healing process of fractures. The plant's impressive ability to alleviate pain and reduce inflammation is well-known. It is incredibly efficient at treating cuts, scrapes, insect bites, burns, and rashes as well.

Parts Used: Leaves and roots

Precautions: Excessive internal use of comfrey can lead to liver damage and potentially harmful carcinogenic effects due to its natural insect-repelling pyrrolizidine alkaloids. Infants and children are particularly vulnerable, so it's important to exercise caution when deciding whether to use comfrey internally or limit it to external applications.

Identifying/Growing: Comfrey, a herbaceous perennial, is originally from Europe but can flourish in areas with partial shade and temperate to warm climates. When fully grown, the plants can reach impressive heights of 3 to 6 feet and widths of 2 to 4 feet.

The flowers of comfrey are beautifully delicate, hanging in clusters that display a range of lovely colors including pink, violet, and cream. The delicate flowers elegantly appear from strong stems decorated with sizable leaves. This plant is quite large, resembling a shrub. However, the stems do not become woody, and the entire plant dies back during winter.

Comfrey is most effectively cultivated through root cuttings, as they offer a simpler and more reliable method of growth in comparison to seeds. Place the cuttings horizontally in the soil, ensuring they are about 3 inches deep and spaced roughly 3 feet apart. It thrives in soil that is rich in nutrients and has plenty of nitrogen.

Regular composting will lead to a plentiful harvest. Once the plants have reached a height of 2 feet, you have the opportunity to harvest the leaves.

Dandelion

Taraxacum officinale

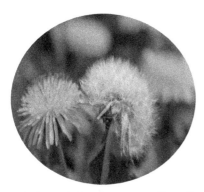

Dandelion is often dismissed as an annoying weed, but its liver detoxifying properties and ability to relieve indigestion, bloating, and constipation make it a valuable addition to your garden. The root possesses medicinal properties, the greens make a nutritious addition to salads, and the fragrant yellow flowers entice pollinators with their nectar.

Parts Used: Roots and sap

Precautions: It is important to be cautious when harvesting dandelions to ensure they have not been exposed to any harmful chemicals like herbicides or pesticides.

Identifying/Growing: The dandelion is easily identifiable with its long, toothy leaves and fluffy, bright yellow flowers. Encouraging dandelions to populate your lawn and garden can be achieved by avoiding the use of herbicides. When harvesting roots and other plant parts, it's important to consider leaving a few plants behind and allowing them to go to seed. This way, you can ensure a bountiful supply of dandelions for the following year.

Echinacea

Echinacea angustifolia, Echinacea purpurea, Echinacea pallida

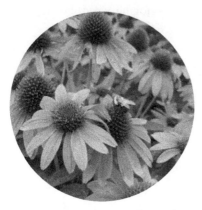

Echinacea is commonly utilized in different remedies for wound care, treating infections, and alleviating cold symptoms. When taken at the first sign of a cold or the flu, you'll notice a decrease in the duration and intensity of symptoms such as coughing, fever, and sore throat. Echinacea possesses impressive antibacterial, antifungal, and antiviral properties, which contribute to its effectiveness in treating various ailments.

Parts Used: Roots

Precautions: Echinacea can potentially interact with pharmaceuticals used in immune system suppression therapy, leading to adverse reactions. It is important to avoid using echinacea if you have a chronic infection like tuberculosis or HIV/AIDS, or if you have an autoimmune disease such as lupus or rheumatoid arthritis. If Echinacea has a negative impact on you, it is advisable to discontinue its use, as it may trigger allergy symptoms in individuals with ragweed allergies.

Identifying/Growing: Echinacea, commonly known as purple coneflower, displays vibrant shades of yellow, orange, and red in the center of its daisy-like flowers.

Although echinacea is naturally found in prairies across North America, it is crucial to be aware of the growing concern of overharvesting. Thus, it is advisable to grow echinacea in your own garden rather than gathering it from its natural habitat.

Echinacea is a breeze to grow in your garden, and not only does it offer remarkable medicinal benefits, it also has the wonderful ability to attract bees and butterflies. This remarkable plant grows to a height of about 4 feet. If allowed to reproduce naturally, it will disperse its seeds and generate new shoots every year. Make sure the plants are placed in a sunny location with well-draining soil that is rich in lime. In return, they will reward you with their stunning beauty and a wide range of affordable solutions.

Fennel

Foeniculum vulgare

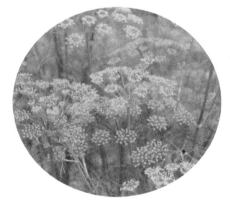

Fennel, known for its pleasant scent that brings to mind licorice, is a widely used ingredient in kitchens worldwide. When used medicinally, the seeds of this product can help alleviate symptoms such as bloating, gas, and abdominal cramps. Fennel has properties that can assist in regulating the female reproductive system, offering relief from symptoms associated with menopause and menstruation.

Parts Used: Seeds

Precautions: Remedies made with seeds and other plant parts are typically safe for use. However, it is advisable to avoid using fennel essential oil if you are pregnant or breastfeeding.

Identifying/Growing: The leaves of fennel are delicate and have a beautiful dark green color. They are accompanied by vibrant green stalks that emerge from the rounded base of the plant. The base itself is ribbed and has a pale greenish-white hue. The stalks reach a maximum height of 5 feet, while the small yellow flowers grow in densely clustered formations.

Fennel thrives in sunny locations and prefers soil that drains well. Plant the seeds 12 inches apart and gently cover them with approximately ¼ inch of soil. Water the planting site gently after seeding, and ensure that the soil remains moist until shoots emerge approximately one to two weeks after planting. To prevent the plants from toppling, it is recommended to stake them once they reach a height of 18 inches.

Collect the seeds once they have turned brown, but before they naturally detach from their umbels. For a smoother process, try using cheesecloth to wrap around the top of the fennel and then cut the stalks. Make sure the seeds are thoroughly dried before placing them in a securely sealed jar.

Feverfew

Tanacetum parthenium

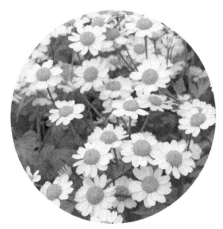

Feverfew offers a soothing and gentle effect that can effectively alleviate the strain and fatigue often associated with headaches. It aids in the prevention of blood platelets from sticking together in the bloodstream and ensures that small capillaries remain unobstructed. Feverfew has been found to be highly effective in preventing and treating migraines.

Parts Used: Leaves

Precautions: Fresh feverfew leaves can cause mouth ulcers. Do not use feverfew during pregnancy and avoid it if you are allergic to ragweed.

Identifying/Growing: Feverfew is a close relative of marigolds and dandelions.
The flowers have small, daisy-like blooms with bright yellow centers and delicate white petals. Growing feverfew is a breeze - just plant the seeds in a sunny area during the spring or summer. When you harvest the plants, it's a good idea to leave some behind and let them go to seed. This way, you can ensure a consistent supply for the following year.

Garlic

Allium sativum

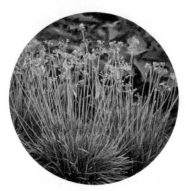

Spicy garlic is an incredibly versatile ingredient that goes beyond its mouthwatering flavor, proving to be a valuable addition in a wide range of recipes. This herb contains over 30 medicinal compounds, including allicin, a potent antimicrobial agent with a broad spectrum of effectiveness. It offers a wide range of health benefits, including the prevention of blood clotting, the reduction of triglycerides and cholesterol levels, and the provision of essential antioxidants.

Parts Used: Roots

Precautions: Overconsumption of garlic can cause gas and heartburn. When used topically, garlic can cause a skin rash in some people with sensitive skin.

Identifying/Growing: Garlic is a breeze to recognize and cultivate, and in numerous regions, you can sow it during the autumn for a bountiful springtime yield, and once more in the early spring for an additional harvest in the fall. Garlic thrives in a sunny location, where the soil has been enriched with nutrient-rich compost. Ensure that the cloves are planted with their tips facing upwards, at a depth of approximately 2 inches, and then apply a generous layer of mulch. It is important to let the soil dry out between waterings to avoid any potential rotting. Additionally, it is recommended to harvest the plant when approximately half of the leaves have turned brown or yellow.

Ginger

Zingiber officinale

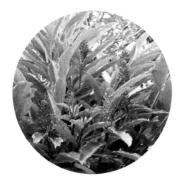

Ginger is an incredibly versatile root that can be used to enhance the flavors of both sweet and savory dishes. Not only is it incredibly tasty, but it also possesses remarkable healing properties that can alleviate a range of discomforts, including cramps and nausea. It possesses natural properties that can assist in thinning the blood and lowering cholesterol levels. Moreover, its remarkable capability to raise body temperature and eliminate toxins has made it a highly sought-after component in remedies for cold and flu.

Parts Used: Roots

Precautions: It is advisable to refrain from consuming ginger if you have a bleeding disorder or gallbladder disease, or if you are currently taking prescription blood thinners, as ginger has blood-thinning properties. When using ginger, it's important to exercise caution if you are pregnant, as it has the potential to stimulate the uterus.

Identifying/Growing: Ginger is a tropical plant that boasts waxy leaves and smooth, fragrant white flowers. When shopping at the grocery store, be sure to choose roots that have a firm texture. If you reside in a tropical climate, ginger can be cultivated outdoors. In colder areas, it can be cultivated in a greenhouse or a sunny indoor spot. For optimal growth, it is recommended to plant the roots in spacious containers, ensuring they are placed at a depth of approximately 10 inches. Ginger plants can reach impressive heights of 4 feet or more, and their blossoms emit a delightful fragrance as a reward for your hard work.

Ginkgo biloba

Ginkgo biloba

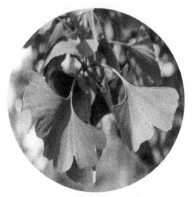

This remarkable deciduous tree features unique fan-shaped leaves. Ginkgo biloba supports healthy blood flow, improves cognitive abilities, sustains energy levels, and may even enhance libido for both men and women. Ginkgo biloba is a great natural choice for effectively managing allergies and asthma because of its antihistamines and anti-inflammatory properties.

Parts Used: Leaves

Precautions: Avoid using ginkgo biloba if you are currently taking prescription monoamine oxidase inhibitor (MAOI) or selective serotonin reuptake inhibitor (SSRI) medications.

It is important to consult with your doctor before using Ginkgo if you are taking prescription blood thinners, as it may enhance their effects.

Identifying/Growing: Ginkgo biloba is renowned for its majestic trees that can soar to heights of up to 100 feet. The leaves of these trees have a unique shape characterized by two lobes. Ginkgo trees boast an astonishing lifespan of over 1,000 years, showcasing their remarkable ability to withstand disease, insects, and pollution. Aside from their practical uses in herbal medicine, these stunning trees can greatly enhance the visual appeal of your home's landscape. Obtain a young tree from a nursery and carefully position it in a prominent spot.

Once the tree reaches maturity, you have the freedom to harvest and make use of its colorful leaves all year round, from spring to fall.

Goldenseal

Hydrastis Canadensis

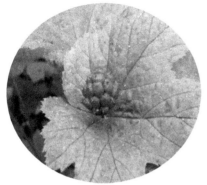

Goldenseal offers significant antiviral and antibacterial advantages due to its abundant hydrastine and berberine content. A versatile herb that can be used for a variety of purposes, goldenseal is often included in remedies for cuts and wounds, sinus infections, respiratory congestion, sore throats, and other common ailments.

Parts Used: Roots, primarily; leaves offer milder benefits

Precautions: Avoid the use of goldenseal if you are currently pregnant or breastfeeding, or if you have been diagnosed with high blood pressure. Goldenseal tincture may lead to stomach irritation, so it is advisable to discontinue internal use if such symptoms arise.

Identifying/Growing: Once, the lush forests from Minnesota to Georgia were home to thriving populations of wild goldenseal. Sadly, the loss of their natural habitat and excessive harvesting have caused a significant decline in their numbers.

These perennial shrubs grow to a maximum height of just 10 inches, with leaves and berries that resemble those of the raspberry. The roots have a thick and knotted appearance, and their interiors are a vibrant shade of yellow.

Growing goldenseal requires a protected area with deep, loamy soil and dappled shade. The rootstock can be divided into sections that are at least ½ inch in size. These sections should be placed about 8 inches apart and buried at a depth of 2 to 3 inches. Make sure to plant the rhizomes during the autumn season and maintain a well-mulched and weed-free area.

Goldenseal has a rather leisurely growth rate and requires up to 2 years to blossom. It typically takes 3 to 4 years for your roots to be ready for harvest.

Hops

Humulus lupulus

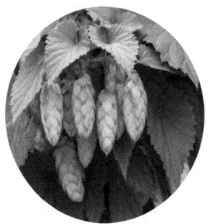

If you've ever experienced a soothing sense of calmness after savoring a beer with a robust hop profile, then you're already acquainted with the impact of hops. Aside from its soothing properties, this herb is recognized for its capacity to alleviate nervous tension and anxiety, aid digestion, and relieve bladder discomfort. Hops have been known to provide relief for menopausal symptoms, such as hot flashes.

Parts Used: Flowers

Precautions: Due to the presence of a powerful plant estrogen called 8-prenylnaringenin, it is not recommended to administer hops to children who have not yet reached puberty, regardless of their gender. Dogs should avoid consuming hops as they can be harmful.

Identifying/Growing: Hops are cultivated on long vines known as bines, which have the remarkable ability to reach lengths exceeding 25 feet. These lush green plants are not commonly found in the wild. They are usually grown by commercial hops growers who use sturdy trellises to support the bines and ensure proper aeration. The medicinal part of hops is the female flower, which has a pale green color and a cone-like shape.

If you have a sunny spot and vertical space for a sturdy trellis capable of supporting at least 25 pounds, then you might have the opportunity to grow hops in your own backyard. It is recommended to grow at least two varieties to ensure cross-pollination, so it's important to plan accordingly.

Plant the rhizomes in spring, once the risk of frost has passed. Make sure to water them regularly and collect the hops once the cones are filled with a rich, golden powder.

Milk thistle

Silybum marianum

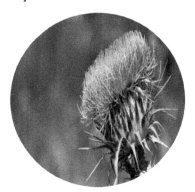

The detoxifying properties of milk thistle have gained significant recognition, extending beyond the realm of herbal medicine. This product features a powerful compound known as silymarin, renowned for its exceptional capacity to rejuvenate liver cells and shield them from detrimental viruses and toxins. If you frequently indulge in alcohol or rely on potent substances, it may be worth considering incorporating milk thistle into your daily regimen.

Parts Used: Seeds

Precautions: Overuse can lead to mild diarrhea

Identifying/Growing: Milk thistles can reach an impressive height of 7 feet. With their large, shiny white-veined leaves, these thistle cultivars are easily distinguishable from others. However, their purple flowers bear a striking resemblance.

It's quite simple to cultivate milk thistle in a wide range of climates. For optimal results, it is recommended to sow the seeds either in early spring or late summer. It is important to ensure that the site is adequately watered, allowing the plants to thrive and grow. Make sure to harvest the seed heads once the flowers have faded, before the wind has a chance to carry the seeds away.

Mullein

Verbascum Thapsus

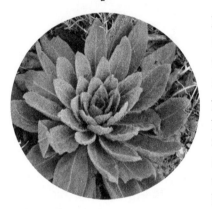

Mullein is a powerful remedy for coughs, earaches, and sore throats, providing both analgesic and antibacterial properties. A homemade poultice created from crushed mullein leaves can serve as an effective remedy for minor wounds, burns, and insect bites.

Parts Used: Leaves and flowers

Precautions: Mullein is generally considered safe. Wildcraft only in areas where you're certain that the soil is free from herbicides, pesticides, and other chemicals.

Identifying/Growing: Mullein is easily recognizable from afar, thanks to its tall central spike adorned with vibrant yellow flowers. These impressive plants typically reach a height of 3 to 4 feet and can be found in various regions including Europe, North America, and the Mediterranean.

Growing your own safe supply of mullein is a straightforward process.

After the flowers fade, it's a good idea to collect seeds from plants. Gently place the seeds onto the soil without burying them, as they require light for germination. Make sure to water the plants and then transplant them once the first leaves start to appear. Harvesting leaves can begin in the first year, while the second year brings forth the flowering spike. Gather the flowers, leaves, and buds from fully grown plants that are two years old, and make sure to leave some plants for natural reseeding in the next year.

Passionflower

Passiflora incarnate

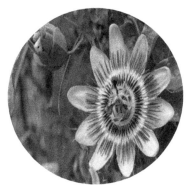

Passionflower is commonly combined with other calming herbs such as valerian and catnip. It acts as a gentle sedative, aiding in sleep when your mind is more active than desired. Passionflower is known for its calming properties, which can be beneficial for reducing anxiety and relieving nerve pain caused by conditions like shingles and neuralgia.

Parts Used: Stems and leaves

Precautions: Because passionflower can cause uterine contractions, it should not be used during pregnancy. Passionflower can increase testosterone and intensify conditions such as baldness and prostate problems when taken in excess.

Identifying/Growing: Passionflower is a robust climbing vine with stunning purple blossoms. It can be found growing wild in certain regions of the southern United States, as well as its native habitats in Central America and Mexico.

Passionflower has the potential to be grown as a perennial plant. Attempting to grow this plant from seed can be quite challenging, as germination is a difficult process. One effective method for propagating passionflower is by taking tip cuttings during the early summer months. Apply liquid rooting hormone to the cuttings and maintain a warm and moist environment until new growth emerges, typically within a span of 2 weeks. Set up a sturdy trellis to support the growth of the passionflower, allowing it to climb and flourish. When the time is right, gather the leaves and stems during the mid- to late summer season.

Peppermint

Mentha piperita

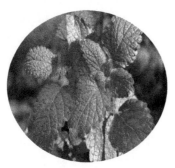

Peppermint is a common ingredient used to add flavors and aromas to products like candy, soap, and toothpaste. This well-known herb is highly effective for addressing digestive issues and provides relief from various discomforts such as body aches, congestion, headaches, and nausea.

Parts Used: Leaves

Precautions: Peppermint can aggravate heartburn. Discontinue use if your digestive problems worsen.

Identifying/Growing: Peppermint can be easily identified by its unmistakable scent. With a vibrant and invigorating presence, it often welcomes you even before you notice the herbs flourishing. Peppermint can be found in various locations, such as near springs, creeks, and ponds.

Peppermint can be grown effortlessly in a pot on your windowsill, or you can opt for a more abundant harvest by cultivating it in your garden. It might be a good idea to allocate a separate container for peppermint, as it has a tendency to spread rapidly and occupy more space than desired if not properly contained. Simply sow the seeds during the spring season, provide them with adequate water, and begin gathering the leaves as they reach maturity.

Raspberry

Rubus idaeus, Rubus strigosus

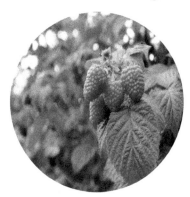

Raspberries are a wonderful addition to a nutritious and wholesome diet. However, it's important not to forget about the leaves when you gather these delectable little fruits. Raspberry leaf is a reliable and secure solution for alleviating symptoms of cold and flu. Teas have been used for centuries to alleviate menstrual discomfort, with a proven track record of success. Raspberry tea can be enjoyed throughout pregnancy as a uterine tonic.

Parts Used: Leaves

Precautions: Although raspberry leaf is safe for the entire family to use, green leaves can cause nausea. Ensure that raspberry leaves are completely dried before use

Identifying/Growing: The raspberry and black raspberry plants can be found growing wild in various locations around the globe, characterized by their thorny canes and toothed, deeply ridged leaves. The flowers come in various colors, such as white, purple, or pink, and eventually transform into green berries. These berries then ripen into tasty morsels, ranging in color from purple to ruby-red. All varieties, whether wildcrafted or cultivated, possess similar medicinal properties.

You can easily acquire raspberry bushes from a nearby nursery and plant them in a sunny location in your garden or yard. Place a protective net over your berries to prevent birds from feasting on them, and collect the leaves as they reach maturity.

Rosemary

Rosmarinus officinalis

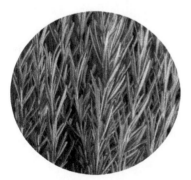

Rosemary, a versatile herb commonly used in cooking, can also provide relief during the cold season. It can be used in comforting soups and teas to alleviate sinus pain.

Rosemary has the ability to enhance circulation and serve as a tonic for the central nervous system. The fragrance enhances cognitive function and focus, while also providing an instant uplift in mood.

Parts Used: Leaves

Precautions: It is important to avoid using this product if you are pregnant or if you have epilepsy. While certain soothing oils have been found to help prevent seizures, others with stronger scents can potentially trigger epileptic incidents.

Identifying/Growing: Rosemary is a small shrub with aromatic, slender leaves and sturdy, woody stems. Delicate blossoms in a range of colors, appearing from late summer onwards.

Although it may be challenging to come across rosemary in its natural habitat, this herb can be easily cultivated in a warm and sunny location. Seeds require a significant amount of time to reach maturity, making it more convenient to consider purchasing plants from a nearby nursery. Collect the leaves in the morning to enhance their flavor and effectiveness.

Sage

Salvia officinalis

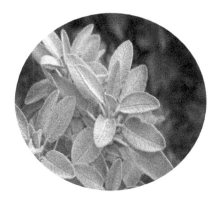

Despite being a widely available and affordable herb, sage is highly effective in treating various health issues such as colds, fevers, hot flashes, painful or heavy periods, rashes, and sore throats. It can also be used to alleviate discomfort in the gums and treat gingivitis. Experience its delightful flavor and enjoy its natural healing properties when used in cooking.

Parts Used: Leaves

Precautions: Sage is generally considered safe

Identifying/Growing: There are approximately 900 different species of Salvia, with some being purely decorative while others have practical uses in cooking and medicine. The elongated, soft leaves have a beautiful silver-green color and are accompanied by lovely pinkish to purplish flowers. The stems are typically woody and upright, with a refreshing aroma that is slightly pungent and tantalizing.

It may take a while for sage to fully mature if grown from seed, but you can easily find mature plants at most nurseries and transplant them into a sunny spot. For optimal results, it's important to consider the specific soil requirements of different sage varieties. Some prefer slightly dry soil, so be sure to check the needs of your plants.

Saw palmetto

Serenoa serrulata

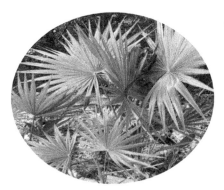

Saw palmetto is widely recognized as a potent herbal remedy for benign prostate hyperplasia, often demonstrating faster results compared to prescribed medications.

Although it may not be widely acknowledged by the mainstream medical establishment in the United States, it is commonly prescribed throughout Europe.

Parts Used: Berries

Precautions: Saw palmetto can be effective in preventing hair loss in men, but it may lead to the growth of unwanted facial hair in women due to its testosterone-boosting properties. Using saw palmetto could potentially exacerbate acne symptoms.

Identifying/Growing: Saw palmetto is native to the US East Coast and can be found from Florida to South Carolina. The trees are short and scrubby, growing no taller than about 10 feet. Fans of spiky leaves give way to oblong berries, which have a reddish-brown color when ripe. The berries should be dried before use in herbal medicines.

Skullcap

Scutellaria lateriflora

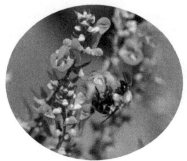

Despite its ominous name, skullcap is a valuable medicinal herb. Skullcap is a natural remedy that provides fast relief from anxiety, nerve pain, and nervous tension. It can also be beneficial in alleviating the discomfort that often comes with menopause.

Parts Used: Stems, leaves, and flowers

Precautions: Avoid using skullcap during pregnancy or while breastfeeding. It is important to avoid the use of skullcap if you have a history of liver disease, epilepsy, or a seizure disorder.

Identifying/Growing: Skullcap is a perennial herb that grows in a creeping manner. The flowers have a range of colors from pale to dark blue or purple, with elongated throats and rounded tops that may bring to mind snapdragons.

Skullcap can be found in damp, partly shady areas across the United States and Europe, making it a fortunate find for wildcrafters. Additionally, cultivating skullcap in your own garden is a simple task. Start by chilling the seeds for a week, and then sow them in pots or flats. Gently press the seeds to ensure they make good contact with the soil, and then give them a light mist of water. Place the container in a warm, sunny spot, such as a windowsill, and cover it with plastic wrap. Take off the plastic wrap once the first green leaves start to show, and remember to lightly mist the young plants every day. Move the seedlings to a location with some shade during the summer and make sure to water them regularly. Make sure to gather the plants when they reach maturity.

St. John's wort

Hypericum perforatum

St. John's wort is a powerful natural remedy that can effectively reduce anxiety and alleviate symptoms of mild depression. Additionally, this herb has powerful antiviral properties that can help reduce the length of time cold sores last when used on the skin. Additional applications involve addressing conditions such as arthritis, fibromyalgia, muscle aches, and sciatica.

Parts Used: Flowers, upper leaves

Precautions: Do not take St. John's wort if you take monoamine oxidase inhibitor (MAOI) or selective serotonin reuptake inhibitor (SSRI) medications

Identifying/Growing: For optimal results, it is recommended to select a high-quality standardized product in capsule form and adhere to the recommended dosage instructions when taking St. John's wort as a dietary supplement. If you are interested in cultivating your own St. John's wort for topical remedies, you will be pleased with the results. These plants are known for their stunning, compact growth and abundant bright yellow blossoms. It thrives in sandy or rocky soil and typically grows to a height of around 2 feet. Once established, St. John's wort is low-maintenance and only requires occasional harvesting of the blooms and upper leaves.

Thyme

Thymus vulgaris

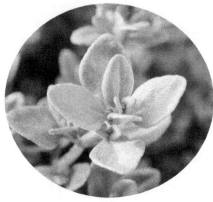

Thyme is a popular herb in kitchens around the world, known for its ability to add a delicious savory taste to dishes. This wonderful herb is a fantastic remedy for colds, providing relief from coughing spasms, chest congestion, and sore throats. It can also help you get a good night's sleep.

Parts Used: Leaves

Precautions: Thyme is generally considered safe, but regular overuse can lead to abnormal menstrual cycles

Identifying/Growing: Thyme has a distinct fragrance that makes it easy to recognize. Delicate oval leaves gracefully adorn slender, woody stems, while tiny pink flowers bloom in the spring and summer. There are approximately 350 different variations of this herb, each with their own unique appearance, but all providing similar medicinal benefits.

Growing thyme can be a breeze, especially if you acquire fully-grown plants and transfer them to a sunny location. This plant thrives in soil that is well-drained and may spread if not properly confined to a pot. You can start collecting the plant tops once the initial spring frost has passed, and cease trimming them approximately one month prior to the arrival of the first frost in the fall.

Consistently harvesting your thyme plants will prevent them from becoming overly woody, while also promoting the growth of fresh and tender leaves for your enjoyment.

Turmeric

Curcuma longa

Turmeric is an exceptional culinary herb known for its delightful, savory flavor. In addition to its culinary applications, it contains curcuminoids and curcurmin, which provide remarkable anti-inflammatory properties. Turmeric offers relief from various painful conditions, such as arthritis, rheumatoid arthritis, and psoriasis.

Parts Used: Root

Precautions: Do not take turmeric in large quantities if you have hypoglycemia. Be careful; the bright yellow color can stain clothing and skin.

Identifying/Growing: Turmeric is a tropical plant that boasts large oval-shaped leaves and vibrant pink flowers. It is originally from India but is extensively grown in Bengal, China, and Java. The rhizomes or roots have a vibrant hue, ranging from yellow to orange or red.

Due to its specific requirements of abundant rainfall and warm temperatures, turmeric can only be grown in tropical climates. If you happen to have a fresh root, you can experiment with growing a plant indoors. Just remember to provide ample water and maintain a minimum temperature of 65 degrees Fahrenheit. It typically takes around 10 months to a year for a new root crop to grow and become ready for harvest.

Valerian

Valeriana officinalis

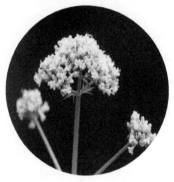

Valerian is often used as a natural sleep aid and can be helpful when combined with other remedies, particularly if pain is interfering with your ability to rest. Although it is powerful and has been likened to valium, it is not addictive. Valerian is also effective in relieving menstrual cramps due to its ability to relax smooth muscles.

Parts Used: Roots

Precautions: Valerian is generally considered safe, but it can act as a stimulant in certain individuals. See how this herb affects you before relying on it for relief from insomnia.

Identifying/Growing: There are various valerian cultivars, each with comparable medicinal effects. The plants have delicate leaves resembling ferns and produce small clusters of flowers in shades ranging from white to pink. These plants can reach heights of 5 feet and bring beauty to your garden, all while offering a bountiful supply of natural medicine.

To successfully grow valerian, it is important to sow the seeds into warm soil once the threat of frost has subsided. Make sure to consistently water your young seedlings, and you'll be pleasantly surprised by the delightful fragrance they emit, reminiscent of vanilla and cinnamon. Collect the roots during the autumn season.

Witch hazel

Hamamelis virginiana

Witch hazel is a gentle and reliable solution for treating acne, cuts and scrapes, insect bites, minor burns, and sunburn. It is suitable for all skin types and has astringent properties that can help reduce swollen veins.

Parts Used: Twigs

Precautions: Witch hazel is generally considered safe.

Identifying/Growing: You can easily find witch hazel at the drugstore, where it is available as a liquid extract among other skin care products. If you're interested in creating your own witch hazel extract, you'll require access to witch hazel trees. These trees can be found in the understory of hardwood forests and they produce vibrant yellow blooms during the winter season, after the leaves have dropped. The leaves have serrated edges and prominent veins. Collect the twigs immediately after the trees bloom to ensure the most potent extract.

Yarrow

Achillea millefolium

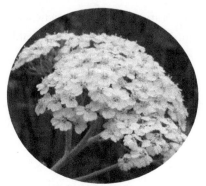

Yarrow delivers a potent medicinal scent and quickly stops bleeding by contracting body tissue and promoting the healing of damaged blood vessels. The "nosebleed plant" promotes clotting and aids in disinfecting minor wounds. Using it in tea or as a tincture helps reduce heavy menstrual bleeding.

Parts Used: Leaves and flowers

Precautions: Avoid consuming yarrow during pregnancy. Some individuals may experience a rash if they have allergies to plants in the Asteraceae family. If any irritation occurs, it is recommended to stop using yarrow.

Identifying/Growing: Yarrow possesses delicate, wispy, silver-green foliage and compact clusters of flowers on sturdy stalks. Wild yarrow typically displays white or pinkish flowers, while certain cultivated varieties may exhibit yellow or bright pink blooms. This herb is found abundantly in North America, Europe, and Asia.

Growing yarrow in your garden proves to be a straightforward task. Plant the seeds and keep them well-watered. Fragrant clusters of leaves will soon give way to beautiful blossoms. Start harvesting this herb once the plants fully grow. Pick the leaves and flowers in the morning and promptly dry them. Yarrow, a self-seeding perennial, allows you to enjoy a bountiful harvest year after year from just one planting.

Conclusion

There are many ways to expand your knowledge of medicinal herbs and how they can be used for natural healing. For example, you might find a local wild crafting class by doing a quick online search.

If you're interested in a more formal approach to education, you may want to consider enrolling in a local herbal medicine program. By engaging in hands-on learning, you can acquire a wealth of practical information. If you don't have access to a herbal medicine program or prefer online courses or conducting your own research, there are other options you can explore.

www.ingramcontent.com/pod-product-compliance
Lightning Source LLC
LaVergne TN
LVHW011554230125
801996LV00012B/401